MEDICAL
MIRACLES

Attributed to Master John Douglas

BOOK ONE

Medical Insights Gained
from Observations of Angelic Reformation

Compelling Stories of
Personal Health Transformations

RICHARD L. SARNAT M.D.

ABOUT THE AUTHOR

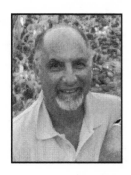 Richard L. Sarnat, MD graduated Phi Beta Kappa from Washington University in St. Louis with a triple focus of philosophy, psychology and premed. He completed his medical degree at Rush Medical College in Chicago and his residency at Northwestern University.

He is a board-certified ophthalmic surgeon and was an early pioneer in the field of co-management between optometrists and ophthalmologists as a population-based solution for under-served areas. He continued to be an innovator in population-based solutions by co-founding Advanced Medicine Integration Group, L.P. (AMI), which contracted with HMO-Illinois, a Blue Cross/Blue Shield company, to form the countries first patient-centered integrative medicine Independent Physicians Association (IPA) in 1999. AMI was also the first company in the USA to obtain waivers from the federal government to allow for the utilization of acupuncture and massage therapy as a covered benefit in the Medicaid population.

Richard was a founding board member of New Chapter Inc., which formulated the nation's first organic food-based vitamin/supplement line and was the largest vitamin/mineral/supplement company in the USA when it sold to Proctor and Gamble in 2012.

He has been a teacher of Transcendental Meditation™ for more than 40 years. He is a graduate of the Elite Development Training Course taught by Master John Douglas.

This book is dedicated
to the memories of
Audri and Jim Lanford
in appreciation for teaching
us all what is possible, and
for giving us the proof
of the Lanford Leap.

ACKNOWLEDGEMENTS

Many people have been instrumental in the writing of this book.

I would like to acknowledge all of my editors: Leslie Elkus, Aaron Frey, Andrew Himmel, Don Sievert PhD, Alexi Teraji John Viviano and Jutta Zimbrich.

I would like to thank my peer review committee: Merrill Galera MD, Philip Lichtenfeld MD, Thomas Tomasselli MD.

Thank you to David Bordow at: david@bordowgraphics.com for my cover and interior design.

Thank you to Bridget Fonger, author of *Superhero of Love: Heal Your Broken Heart & Then Go Save the World,* for our website development: medicalmiracle.info

TABLE OF CONTENTS

MEDICAL DISCLAIMER

To aid with the launch of this book, and the dissemination of the knowledge contained in this book, I and other scientifically-minded individuals have founded a non-profit LLC, the STS Foundation. "STS" is short for Science, Technology and Spirituality. **I am but a spokesman on behalf of the Foundation and wish to remind the reader that this book and my observations are not to be taken as medical advice from a physician. Rather, my words are to be taken from the perspective of a medically trained observer, vouching for the validity and reproducibility of this specific opportunity for faith-based healing via the knowledge presented by Master John Douglas, and the Church of the Master Angels (CMA).**

PROLOGUE

Towards the end of this book there is a question and answer session, which is my attempt to satisfy all questions that were raised during the review process by my medical peers and other critical thinkers.

However, I believe there is one question from them that should be addressed even at the beginning of the book: **"Why did you write this book and what do you hope it achieves, especially when there is a high likelihood of being ridiculed by your own medical profession?"**

I feel that this is a very fair question to ask. And, I want you, the reader, to hear my answer before you commit your time and effort to read this book.

The questioner is correct. I do expect a lot of professional ridicule. That being said, I am at peace with the fact that I can't really control how the book is received and have no clue as to what will be achieved by its publication.

What I do know, is that I view my role primarily as that of a medical historian, attempting to understand and give context to the empirical reality and observations that I have had the privilege to witness over the last ten years.

Quite honestly, this attempt on my part to make sense of all that I have witnessed is a shared journey for us both. My understanding of the complexities and enormity of these observations has changed not merely my thinking about how the universe works, but more importantly, how

I should live my life and properly interact with all that I see by knowing who I am and what is my place in the universe.

That, I guess, is my goal. There certainly is no other material metric of success that comes to mind.

1

Sarcoidosis–Curing the Incurable Disease

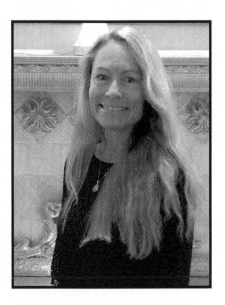

Imagine that you are living with a constant pain of seven out of ten to ten out of ten, 24 hours a day, for more than three years.

Imagine that have been told that your disease is incurable.

Imagine that this disease creates small tumors, called granulomas, which can form anywhere in your body–eyes, heart, lungs, muscles, nerves and internal organs.

Imagine that you have been treated with steroids and opioids and nothing relieves your pain, which you describe "as if I was constantly being bitten by red ants."

Imagine that this process is beginning to affect your heart muscles and you know that future heart surgery is looming ever closer.

Then, one day, you have the realization that nothing in the world of conventional medicine will provide a cure and **that to survive, you must now find a miracle.**

This is the story of Jan who was diagnosed with the rare and "incurable" autoimmune disease of Sarcoidosis in 2012, when both of her legs swelled up "and looked like elephant legs."

Her symptoms progressed so that "the pain was intense, ranging from pressure in the chest, to deep bone ache, to throbbing unrelenting pain in all swollen areas."

Her diagnosis of the autoimmune disease sarcoidosis was never in question. She had seen many, many specialists and had all the classic lab abnormalities seen in sarcoid patients.

Luckily, she found her miracle.

Her miracle was delivered in the form of an Australian gentleman by the name of Master John Douglas. He is a most humble and unassuming person. A master of self-deprecating and off-color Australian humor, he often describes himself as, "balding, overweight and missing my opportunity to be an underwear model. Nature has given me the most unlikely wrapping for the message I must deliver."

Regardless of his first appearances, Master John has a successful track record of performing miracles. He is known for curing the "incurable." He was born with clairvoyant senses beyond the common man and has dedicate his life to cultivating the ability to doing medical miracles.

It is hard for us to appreciate what it must be like to have a sense of smell like a dog, x-ray vision like Superman or heightened senses like Spiderman, but that is the world Master John lives in.

At present, conventional medicine does not have a cure for sarcoidosis, as current medical science believes that the body literally attacks itself in a disease process termed "autoimmune." Master John literally looked into Jan's blood cells, like Superman with x-ray vision, and discovered that "her blood cells just did not look normal."

He saw "two nano-sized bacteria within a single white blood cell" and in his experience this phenomenon had never been seen before. He then concluded that, "this would only occur in a pathological situation."

The proof was in the pudding, as they say. Within seconds of Master John invoking the celestial realm of the Master Healing Angels for a cure, all of Jan's pain immediately and completely disappeared. She remains pain-free to this day, four years later.

Of scientific interest, all of her initial laboratory findings, which were typical of sarcoidosis, now have returned to normal as well.

So how do we try to make sense of this rather amazing story of a well-documented incurable disease that now has clinically been cured?

Is Jan the victim of mind control, a hallucination or placebo?

Or, is there a logical explanation for not only this

miraculous healing but the many thousands of similar stories, testimonials and even peer-reviewed medical case studies which all point to the fact that medical miracles attributed to Master John Douglas now occur with great precision, specificity and regularity?

Before we tackle this question head-on, or present another story of miraculous healing, perhaps a short detour to part of a previously published interview with Master John Douglas, written by Amber Terrrell, will be illuminating.

2

Excerpts from an Interview with Australian Healer, Master John Douglas

When he was just nine years old, John Douglas had a spontaneous clairvoyant awakening that allowed him to see pretty much everything–what people were thinking and feeling, what emotional and psychological baggage they were lugging around, what unresolved karmic issues were impacting them or would later impact them, and what effect negative energy such as fear and stress has upon health and the environment–just for starters. Quite a load for a nine-year-old!

We don't know how many children there may have been whose perceptions opened up in similar ways and were given medicines to help them be "normal" or possibly even sent away to an institution to be "cured." Fortunately, John was born into a spiritually mature family who helped him to understand and embrace his gifts. As a teenager, growing up in Australia, his abilities continued to develop through a powerful connection with angelic beings and Celestial Masters who began to guide him to develop and use his gifts for the benefit of humanity. His mission: "To repair and develop the spirit in order to heal and positively evolve the spirit and physical body so greatness and fulfillment of one's life mission can be realized."

We asked John to talk about the unique nature of his abilities and his work.

Q: *Your mission sounds like a huge undertaking. How do you go about accomplishing something like that in a practical way?*

John: For me, the evolution of mankind is the path, the dharma and the mission. I'm just somebody who had a vehicle that was right to be used by Nature. I'm not a scientist. I'm not a philosopher or a guru. But I have a unique view on the nature of our reality. I live it every day, just as you live your daily life. At the age of nine the frequency of my vision expanded to enable me to view the nature of reality, to view the entire realm clearly, just as you are seeing me now. And what I see is, everything is frequency. Your thoughts, emotions, desires, weaknesses, beliefs, karmic governance–all of these things are energies, composed of particular, identifiable frequencies. Just imagine if you had a giant radio tuner that can detect all of these different frequencies, at will. That is essentially what I have, and it has allowed me to analyze and discover and experiment and find the real causes of disease in the body.

3

"Everything is Frequency"

According to Master John Douglas, "everything is frequency" and he experiences life different from us. He calls himself a "giant radio tuner."

Granted, this is not the way that the common man describes his experience of the world. But oddly enough, this description is almost identical to the viewpoint of some of the world's greatest scientists. To quote a few of history's greatest minds.

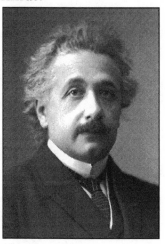

"Everything is energy and that's all there is. Match the frequency of the reality you want, and you cannot help but get that reality. It can be no other way. This is not philosophy, this is physics."
Albert Einstein

"Future medicine will be the medicine of frequencies." Albert Einstein

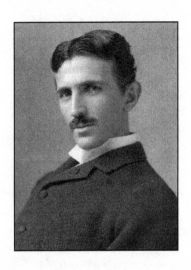

"If you want to find the secrets of the universe, think in terms of energy, frequency and vibration."
Nikola Tesla

Today, almost all innovators and scientists talk about the world in terms of "frequencies." According to quantum physics, all matter emits light in frequency.

It took me awhile to reconcile the difference between how Master John Douglas views the world and how modern medicine views the world. But I now believe that the two viewpoints are completely compatible. They simply emphasize different aspects of reality. Let me explain by using this example.

Modern medicine categorizes infectious organisms, such as bacteria, viruses, parasites, etc. by their morphology (how they look) and by their DNA.

Master John Douglas categorizes and recognizes the entire universe of infectious organisms by the emanation of their individual frequencies. Using frequency to categorize infectious life forms enables him to discover a world of infectious organisms which is currently unknown to medical science. If Einstein is correct, then Master John's categorization of the universe into the study of frequencies may well unlock the future of our ability to survive as we go forward on this planet in an era of antibiotic resistance. And in case you have not read the news lately, this growing era of antibiotic resistance is truly perilous.

According to the United States Governments Center for Disease Control in Atlanta, Georgia, each year, at least two million people in the U.S. become infected with bacteria that are resistant to antibiotics and at least 23,000 people die each year as a direct result of these infections.

It is not that either system of categorization or how we gain knowledge is wrong. Modern medicine has brought us a long way from the pre-antibiotic era of shortened lifespans due to infectious diseases. However, I believe that this post-antibiotic era, with superbugs, flesh eating bacteria and the untamed growth of chronic diseases, requires a new and innovative non-antibiotic solution. Could it be that this solution is unlocked by the study of frequencies, as so many great scientists suggest?

I think we will find that to be true. But don't take my word for it. Keep reading and decide for yourself.

4

Myocardial Infarction
(also known as a Heart Attack)

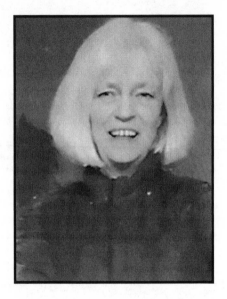

I am choosing to present this case early in the book because we might as well come to grips with the fact that the angelic kingdom exists and that some of us, who are very lucky, can see and hear this kingdom, not much differently from "looking at the leaves on trees."

Depending on which survey you read, 80% or more of all people living in the USA believe in the existence of angels. I certainly have reason to believe in the existence of the celestial realm and if you don't, perhaps this story will help change your mind.

Kathryn, the subject of our story, is a 66-year-old white female who has been practicing Transcendental Meditation™ for 48 years. While she was probably born with some level of clairvoyance, her longstanding practice of meditation has refined her ability to see and hear the celestial world of angels.

Three weeks before her impending cardiac event, Kathryn tells the story that while she was fully awake, in a normal state of consciousness, "a large angel would appear to me and ask me if I was interested in accepting a new assignment. In other words, leaving this body/incarnation and reincarnating elsewhere. This angel appeared to me on three separate occasions with the same message." She relates to me that, "I did not answer the angel directly but remembers that her attitude was one of being open to however life unfolded."

The Sunday morning of her cardiac event, Kathryn remembers sitting at her kitchen table after breakfast reading emails. Suddenly, she experienced a strange cramp emanating from her heart and spreading throughout her central core. This "cramp" then progressed to include both her arms and legs. At that point, she lost all muscle control and fell off of her chair onto the kitchen floor. She also remembers having left jaw pain at this time.

Luckily, her telephone was in reach of where she had collapsed. She was able to call 911 and crawl on the floor, "GI Joe style" to open the front door for the paramedics. While crumpled on the floor, she also had the presence of mind to send an emergency text describing her medical situation to Master John Douglas, as well as to other close friends who were very familiar with his healing techniques.

These friends initiated a Silent Faith Remote (SFR) healing, which is available twenty-four hours per day, seven days per week, at the Church of the Master Angels website (www.masterangels.org), in order to reach Master John. She also remembers requesting help from the angelic kingdom, while incapacitated on the kitchen floor.

By the time she and the paramedics arrived at the local emergency room, her dizziness and left jaw pain still persisted but she was now able to ambulate. At the local emergency room, an EKG of her heart, along with blood work, was done. Her results were highly suggestive of an acute myocardial infarction, also known as a heart attack. She was sent by ambulance to a regional university affiliated medical center for further evaluation and treatment.

The university medical center admitted her to a cardiac telemetry ward for additional blood work and cardiac monitoring overnight, while she awaited a cardiac catheterization known as an angiogram, on Monday morning.

She surprised her new cardiologist when the Monday morning EKG and angiogram were both found to be normal. This was not the expectation initially given to our patient. Her invasive cardiologist had led her to believe that "I had a 95% chance of needing a stent and would probably be taking two different cardiac pharmaceuticals for the rest of my life."

After her angiogram, her invasive cardiologist told

her that, "I am completely mystified by what actually happened." He also told her that, "it made no medical sense that her angiogram is now normal."

Interestingly, after her full recovery, the angel who had visited her three times prior to the cardiac event again "spoke" to her. Kathryn was "concerned whether my decision to stay in this body at this time would be problematical in the larger view of things."

The angel communicated to her that, "my decision to stay is not a problem at all, as the realm that I would have been assigned to has a very different experience of time. No matter how long I live on earth," she was told, "it would be like showing up to work only twenty seconds late for my new assignment."

So, how do we make sense of what happened? By definition, an elevated troponin blood level means that damage to her heart muscle has already occurred and this typically occurs only when significant pathology will be found on her angiogram.

How could an experienced cardiologist, who believed her patient would require both a stent and life-long medication be so wrong?

Welcome to the world of medical miracles, where the unthinkable and unknown become almost routine, in my experience, having watched hundreds, if not thousands of similar cases.

Let's reconstruct the timeline from the moment Kathryn collapsed at the kitchen table to the time her angiogram was read as normal. If we could do so, we would find that by direct angelic intention and intervention, a blood clot that had been clinically significant enough to produce laboratory evidence of an acute heart attack and cause her to collapse to the floor, was dissolved and harmlessly relocated to the spleen. The spleen acts as a filter to remove potentially harmful blood clots, which otherwise can cause strokes and heart attacks.

How can I be so sure that this version of the story timeline actually occurred and that it was not just luck or placebo that prevented further damage?

To understand that answer, we must peel back the onion a few layers, and delve deeper into why medical miracles are already quite evident on a daily basis and will soon be commonplace and understood scientifically.

5

Come on Doc! Miracles, Angels and Prayer!! Really?

Before we go any further, I think it is a perfectly legitimate question to ask: "How and why is a conventionally trained medical doctor, like yourself, involved with the study of medical miracles, celestial angels and measuring pranic frequencies (Master John's description) of the spiritual bodies?"

I guess the short answer is that I have never been uncomfortable trying to make sense of the conflicting views which are presented by competing hypotheses within the realm of science. It was most unusual for a premed student to major in philosophy. It was even more unusual that a budding physician would be attracted to learning Transcendental Meditation, Hatha Yoga and Tai Chi and continue with those practices for almost 45 years.

While in medical school, a number of other students and I arranged for a private tutor and private classes in Traditional Chinese Medicine, learning acupuncture and acupressure along the way. In the pursuit of finding all possible options to aid with the healing process, I sought out the additional knowledge and differing perspectives of homeopathy, chiropractic, naturopathy, herbal medicine and even energy medicine.

I have always looked at the world around me with open eyes, ignoring the narrative which society tells us is "the truth" and researching my own assessment of "the truth of our collective reality."

This often proved very useful in both my personal life and my medical career. I jumped on the bandwagon of the Natural Foods industry, and the value of nutrition both for prevention and treatment, long before my medical colleagues.

I was treating macular degeneration by nutritional supplementation before the national trials proving its efficacy were even imagined. Nutritional strategies are now the standard of care for the prevention of macular degeneration.

In 1997 I co-founded what I believe was the nation's first patient-centered integrative medical delivery system in a managed care setting contracted with HMO-Illinois, a Blue Cross and Blue Shield company. While it was common sense to believe that it is more cost effective and clinically effective to create a health care system that focuses on wellness and prevention and relegate pharmaceuticals, surgery and medical devices to secondary and tertiary care options, until AMI, no one had ever constructed a clinical trial to test this hypothesis in the real world.

This same patient-centric integrative health model, according to its strategic national plan, is the future health care delivery system of the Veterans Administration. It is also the current preferred interdisciplinary model for the treatment of chronic pain, according to recent publications from the *Institute of Medicine* and the *Journal of Family Practice.*

So, is it a stretch in our current health care system to entertain a serious discussion of the validity of medical miracles?

Absolutely!!

Is it an important discussion to pursue?

Absolutely!!

Is invoking celestial angelic help to kill a world of unseen and unknown infectious life forms, which exist outside of our current scientific knowledge, an uncomfortable discussion for a scientist to have?

Absolutely!!

But no more uncomfortable than it was historically for those original scientific pioneers who hypothesized "the germ theory" prior to widespread use of the microscope and the visualization and verification of this hidden world of infectious microbes.

The original scientists and proponents of the germ theory were ridiculed for washing their hands and believing that unseen microbes were the root cause of disease.

The more things change, the more they seem the same.

Or, as is often said, those who forget history are doomed to repeat it.

So, let's be fearless in our pursuit of truth and bold enough to discuss another medical miracle.

6

Cancer

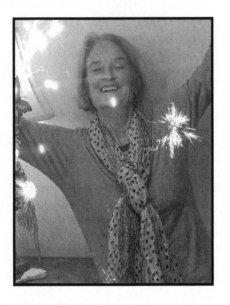

I have heard Master John say that for a healer to be taken seriously, they must be able to cure that scourge of our time–cancer.

Master John would be the first to say, that he is not 100% successful in being able to cure all cancers, in all people, at this time. Why can certain diseases can be healed and others not? Why can certain individuals can be healed and others not? Later in the book we will talk about why that is so.

But, I do remember his excitement, when he had one of his first instantaneous cures of a stage-four cancer, which was visible, at least to him clairvoyantly, in real-time.

Our subject, Ann, is a 65-year-old white female who first discovered she had **"biopsy proven invasive squamous cell carcinoma of the anus" in 2008.** The details of this case have already been published in a peer-reviewed medical journal and can be easily accessed by hitting the tab called "research" located at the top of the home page on the CMA website at www.masterangels.org. This published article and other published articles will drop down from the research tab, for those who wish to know all of the scientific details.

For those of us who prefer the abbreviated version of the story, suffice it to say that in the patient's chart, her Oncologist wrote: "...**the chance of cure is small to none.**"

These are probably the words that bring the most dread to anyone of us. They usually foretell the short horizon of our own mortality.

Luckily on July 8th, 2010 Ann received a miracle. This was the day she first encountered Master John Douglas. Ann describes this encounter as: "I was feeling very light as I was sitting within the energy aura of Master John Douglas, which felt like sitting in a candle-lit circle filled with peace, innocence, protection, love and a state of simplicity where all worries were gone. I felt the presence of Angelic Beings in the room cradling me and sprinkling sparks of stardust inside me. Suddenly, I felt a 'snap' in my lower belly and chest and watched and allowed an oily vapor to come out of me and dissipate into the air."

On the other side of the equation, Master John Douglas reports that: "I remember that this person was a faithful, kind and gentle person, who showed no cynicism or doubts about her potential to be healed. The moment that we met together during the five-minute personalized healing session, I could directly and clairvoyantly view the cancerous cells and proceeded to apply the Angelic Reformation to her physiology on a molecular level. Due to her spiritual worthiness, what ensued was remarkable. The cells that were cancerous literally reformed before my eyes and all energetic structures of the cancerous cells were expelled and instantly replaced by healthy structures. As always, being cautious, I wished her well, and told her that she had received a very special healing that many had not received previously. She was in awe, so I knew she experienced something profound."

A few months after the healing session described above, re-staging scans ordered by a new Oncologist showed no evidence of her former metastatic disease. Ann remained in full remission until her disease reoccurred in January of 2013. Ann is still active in her chosen profession and alive today.

Now wait a minute you may protest, incredulous, that I am presenting a supposed miracle, when the patient has had a relapse after less than four years. I would encourage you to enjoy the miracle for what it is: the complete, spontaneous remission of a stage-four cancer. This is a remission which the patient experienced in real-time as a metamorphosis of sorts ("an oily vapor dissipated into the air") and that the healer simultaneously experienced in real-time ("The cells that were cancerous literally reformed before my eyes and all energetic structures of the cancerous cells were expelled and instantly replaced by healthy structures").

Why did Ann receive this miracle healing?

Master John leaves no doubt as to why: **"Due to her spiritual worthiness what ensued was remarkable."**

There are so many variables to consider:

a. The worthiness of the patient.

b. The skill of the healer.

c. The celestial angels that act as intermediaries.

d. Why do bad things happen to good people to begin with?

e. Why do good people experience a miracle only to suffer a relapse eventually?

f. What does the present state of medicine have to say about infectious organisms as the cause of cancer?

If you are starting to get the idea that the more you know, the more questions you will have, or that our current understanding of medicine now seems very limited, welcome to my world.

For you see, we are really on a journey of discovery. It is a journey we are taking together in real-time as we say.

I don't pretend to have all the answers. I don't pretend to even know all the questions that should be asked. All I know is that for ten years, I have witnessed directly or indirectly, thousands of medical miracles which defy current scientific medical explanations.

As a medical professional acting more like a medical historian, attempting to document what I have been privileged to witness, all I can do is take you on this journey with me in the hopes that together we will arrive at a better understanding of reality than if I take this journey alone.

So how do I keep my sanity and try to make sense of all of this when even my mom, not the most flexible thinker at age 89, will think I am crazy when she reads this book?

Good question; and one that I am not sure I have a ready-made answer for yet.

Let's see if we can get some plausible answers to our many questions beginning with Chapter 7.

7

How and Why Miracles are Now Predictable Daily Events

Master John Douglas has often said that: "…he exists half in this earthly realm and half in the celestial realm, simultaneously." If his assertion is true, what does this really mean?

While I admit that I could be wrong, my understanding of this statement is that Master John Douglas is active on this planet as the human incarnation of a Celestial Being. For those of us who are keeping track, this is not an unusual event. I believe that most of history's great spiritual teachers fall into the same category.

It is my belief that most great spiritual leaders have arrived on earth at a specific point in time and space to deliver new knowledge and ideas, which were necessary at that exact historical moment in time.

It is my belief that we, as humans, are on a path of ascension towards the ultimate knowledge of who we are, to better know our place in the universe, and to fully know our God.

For a Celestial Being to voluntarily come to earth would be the opposite. They would be on a path of descension, in order to fully experience the human condition, and to deliver whatever packet of knowledge is required at that time.

If we hypothesize that Master John Douglas has incarnated as a human being, yet is simultaneously a Celestial Being, and that his enhanced sensory mechanisms are abilities that transcend normal human capabilities, it suddenly becomes a logical possibility why someone with no formal conventional medical training is able to create miraculous healings and medical remissions across such a variety of poorly understood diseases.

Master John Douglas reports that: "I was born with a complement of 19 clairvoyant senses." He then refined them during a lifetime of practice and discipline. In his formative years he actually entered a monastery for a number of years to receive instruction on the training of his clairvoyant senses. He is able to use these enhanced senses to discover the hidden Laws of Nature, which are the cause and effect of all things, including health and illness.

For example, his sense of sight is analogous to having a real-time combination light microscope and electron microscope. Master John directly visualizes the atoms, molecules and cells in our physical body, "like I see the leaves on trees." By invoking the Master Healing Angels and requesting the intervention of the Divine, Master John seems to be able to instantaneously, and with intention, to reorder both the atomic and molecular levels within the physical structures of our physiology to relieve the pain and suffering of a given ailment. While I am restricting this discussion primarily to medicine and science, these same abilities can be used to unlock all of the hidden Laws of Nature which govern all spheres of life.

Most importantly, the case studies reported herein, are not an historical retrospective of random miracles that have occurred to worthy individuals deserving of special spiritual blessing, as has been documented historically in the theological mystical literature describing the lives of many Saints. The case studies presented here are the evidence of deliberate and scientifically verifiable miraculous healings and medical remissions, where the mechanisms of action are not only revealed but are taught and can be replicated by the general human population–by those of us who work with Master John Douglas's tools, attend his seminars and take the Elite Development Course.

So now we have another new wrinkle in the story. What is the Elite Development Course?

Is Master John really able to teach the common man how to perform medical miracles?

Will graduates of this course have healing abilities equal to Master John Douglas?

I promise to answer all of these questions and more before our journey ends. But for now, let's go to another example of a medical miracle.

8

Let's Not Forget Our Furry Friends

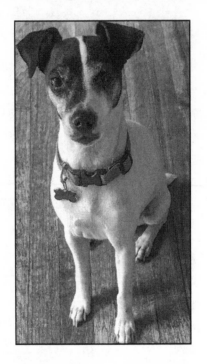

Miah is a 6-year-old Jack Russell Terrier who began showing signs of a severe systemic infection on September 2, 2017. At that time, she had uncontrolled vomiting, which was described as "white and foamy", and extreme watery diarrhea which was bloody and foul smelling. A phone call was made to the Miah's Veterinarian who said that, "it might be Parvo, even though the dog had received a Parvo immunization shot less than three years ago."

Nancy, the owner of the dog happened to be an Elite Development Course graduate and immediately scanned Miah for the frequency of the Parvovirus. Nancy found that Miah did, in fact, have a mutated, hybrid form of Parvovirus, which explains why the dog was susceptible to reinfection. The Parvo had now mutated into a hybrid form, thus making it active even during the protected duration of her previous vaccination. Believing that she had discovered the root cause of Miah's distress, Nancy began to do healing requests with the Master Healing Angels to eradicate the virus. As Parvo is lethal, simultaneously, she requested a Silent Faith Remote with Master John on the CMA website: "Just to leave no stone unturned."

Prior to the healing requests, Miah had been vomiting uncontrollably every five minutes. Yet within thirty minutes of invoking the healing requests with the Master Healing Angels, and by the time that Miah was brought to the Vet's office, she presented to the Vet looking completely normal and energetic. While the Vet's suspicion of Parvo was now reduced given the energetic presentation of Miah, for the sake of completeness, he decided to do a Parvo screen. The Parvo screen was still positive.

Miah's owner was told by the Veterinarian: "If the dog could survive the next five days of symptoms, then chances are good that she would survive long term."

Miraculously, after Nancy's healing requests to the Master Healing Angels via the Silent Faith Remote healing placed on the CMA website, Miah's former symptoms of vomiting and diarrhea completely resolved. Her owner gradually introduced her to a normal diet. Within two days, she became energetic, alert and happy and has been that way ever since.

Parvo is a devastating event, because it is potentially fatal and because it is exceptionally contagious. I have been a board member at my local no-kill animal shelter for over 15 years. I can attest to the fear and death a Parvo epidemic creates within a local animal shelter. Imagine how many furry lives can be saved and countless man/women-hours saved by avoiding the labor-intensive quarantine measures required to stabilize a Parvo infected environment. A single Silent Faith Remote healing can save an individual animal and an entire shelter from such a fate.

This case study is also unique in that it is our only report of a non-human miraculous healing. In my experience as a pet owner, animals react to miraculous healing requests even faster than humans. My theory is that they have less subconscious baggage and socialized constructed complexity to block their innocent reception to Divine Grace. Scientifically, one could also argue that animal healing removes any placebo affect from the equation.

9

Peripheral Neuropathy with Chronic Foot Drop

One of my buddies, who we will call Dave, and whom is a major personal injury attorney nationwide, once said that, "A foot drop case is money in the bank. They never get better."

This foot drop case, of course, is the exception to that rule.

Our patient, a 65-year-old white female who we will fictitiously call Karen, originally met Master John Douglas in 2009, when she attended a public-seminar that Master John offered during that timeframe. Since 2009, she reports using many of his audio Health Repair tools on a daily basis, along with her daily practice of Transcendental Meditation.

In 2015, she first noticed that her right foot developed a subtle foot drop. Her foot would "flop" as she walked. She also noticed "a definite loss of control in her foot" at this time. She was seen by her Internist, who made the diagnosis of peripheral neuropathy with a right foot drop.

Her symptoms became worse over time. She further reported "losing the natural roll of my ankle as I walked and what was a subtle flop, now became a heavy thud of the foot."

Given this worsening progression of her symptoms, she

was referred to a Neurologist. When he asked her to walk across the room on her heels, she was unable to do so. Her Neurologist then referred her to outpatient physical therapy, which she reports "helped me overall but did not help my foot drop at all."

In 2017, she attended a Master John Douglas public seminar where she was able to see Master John Douglas for a five-minute private session. She told him of her diagnosis and longstanding foot drop. After a few moments of clairvoyantly looking at her body, she reports that: "Master John burst out laughing and said that she did not have a peripheral neuropathy at all. She had a specific type of bacteria which has a predilection for the lower extremities of the body. These bacteria often create small blood clots which then cause symptoms such as your foot drop."

She reports that Master John said: "I will invoke the Master Healing Angels to kill the bacteria and remove all the blood clots now." After he did this, she reports that: "I immediately felt a rushing flow of blood to my right foot, which although not blue, was never the same color as my left foot. I experienced an immediate change of color and delightful warmth within my foot, which now resembled the color and feel of the other foot."

She remembers thanking Master John, and then to prove to herself that she was fully healed, she demonstrated to him that she was able to walk out of the room on her heels without difficulty.

The function of her right foot has remained stable since the day of that miraculous healing in 2017.

Well Dave, you cannot win them all.

Yet again, we see a totally unexpected outcome from the standpoint of current medical thinking and expectations. Both her Internist and her Neurologist believed that her foot drop was secondary to a diabetic peripheral neuropathy. The natural course of a foot drop secondary to a diabetic peripheral neuropathy is that it rarely, if ever, improves, especially after the foot drop has become chronic, as it was in this case, lasting two and a half years before resolution. This is because conventional medicine does not currently have treatments which reverse long standing neurological damage.

It would never have occurred to either physician that an infectious bug would be the root cause of her foot drop. And while the skeptical reader, especially a professional in the medical field, might ascribe her sudden recovery to placebo, I assert that this is even more far-fetched than understanding that the root cause was an unknown infection creating a hyper-viscosity syndrome.

Like most of our case studies, the diagnostic process of identification of the infectious agent, killing of the infectious agent, and the immediate reversal of symptoms, suggests a cause and effect relationship that underlies her recovery.

In fact, the astounding rapidity of her recovery to full function within minutes is easier to understand if the mechanism of recovery was the removal of a blood clot and the restoration of adequate blood flow versus the immediate healing of a focal and chronic nerve degeneration. Just some academic food for thought for the anatomists and physiologists who might be reading this book.

In other words, from a structure/function standpoint, which is how we look at these things in medicine, my explanation of events, even though it invokes the realm of angelic celestial help, actually makes more physiological sense than any other alternative explanation.

Similar to many of our other case study subjects, experiencing her own miraculous healing inspired Karen to take the Elite Development Course in 2018. She excitedly remembers the very first time she was able to verify her own healing abilities with the following story: "Three months before taking the Elite Development Course, I had a penny-sized red lesion on my right forearm. This lesion was unresponsive to the antifungal cream given to me by my primary care doctor. As soon as I learned to scan at the course, I found a "mutated alien fungus" living within the lesion. Within seconds of my invocation to the Master Healing Angels to help heal this lesion and kill this specific infectious agent, the lesion resolved entirely–right before my eyes! I guess conventional antifungal creams kill only earthly fungus, not mutated alien fungus."

Ok, so this brings us back to discussing the Elite Development Course and how ordinary folks like us are given the tools invoke the help of the Master Healing Angels to obtain their own medical miracles.

10

The Elite Development Course

When I first met Master John Douglas about ten years ago, he was helping people on a one-on-one basis, doing personal sessions that typically lasted an hour. At that time, he decided that to successfully fulfill his mission, he was going to have to expand his abilities in order to reach more people simultaneously. As such, I was lucky enough to be present at his first ever public seminar.

While at this seminar, I remember that Master John was asked by a member of the audience, whether he could, or would, teach people how to heal each other, similar to what he does? At first, he said: "No, I will not be able to teach others." But then, a funny look came over his face, as if he had changed his mind, He then said that: "Maybe at some time in the distant future teaching people will be possible, but not right now."

Now fast forward to August of 2013 and the first Elite Development Course. Master John taught 50 people the basics of how to develop their own abilities to obtain healings. Here is what I and the other course participants experienced.

1. **Master John upgraded our physical, human central nervous systems to become more like divine, celestial central nervous systems.**

2. He attuned our conscious mind to be able to discern the different frequencies within each particle of creation. Master John says that this was like turning us into cosmic radio tuners.

3. With our new, more deeply silent and blissful mind, we were given a more direct communication link to the celestial realm of the Master Healing Angels.

4. Now, imagine if every human being on Earth took the Elite Development Course. These abilities, which are latent in everybody, would allow everyone to be directly linked to the celestial realm of the Master Healing Angels. Daily "miracles" would become almost commonplace.

5. As our direct link to the celestial realm of creation grows even more with the regular use of this technology, we will find that our ability to know our God, and our place in the universe, will grow as well. We spontaneously will begin to live our lives much more closely attuned to the Divine pulse of all creation.

While you may think that the points listed above are a hard sell, if anything, they barely scratch the surface of the total transformation of mind, body and spirit that occurs at the Elite Development Course.

As Master John always says: "How much proof do people need? Who else can teach you how to kill a virus, a parasite, molds, yeast and fungus? Who else can give you the knowledge and power to protect your family and friends from the future horrors of the microbial world, like flesh eating bacteria? Who else in the recorded annals of history has ever performed this many scientifically documented miracles?"

The short answer: no one that I am aware of.

The Elite Development Course is now an annual event. Applications to attend this course are available to the public on the CMA website. The caveat is that Master John has publicly said numerous times that acceptance to attend the Elite Development Course is not predicated on any earthly criteria. He asserts that it is the Master Healing Angels who decide which applicant is ready to attend or not.

The Elite Development Course occurs on multiple weekends every August. Each separate course is taught over a four-day weekend. Master John enables each course participant to develop the art of "scanning/divining", a consciousness-based skill whereby the course participant is able to measure the unique and individual frequencies emanating from all particles in creation. Or, as he puts it, "I will teach you how to hear the song of every particle in creation."

The basis of this ability is an actual physical, emotional, and spiritual transformation of the course participant's physiology and consciousness. Our limited human perspective is transformed into a cosmic, angelic perspective.

This transformation on the level of physiology and consciousness is what Master John calls an "Angelic Reformation." This reformation occurs in all course participants and is the foundation of these developing abilities. Each course participant develops a more cosmic, multi-dimensional, multi-pointed awareness.

Maybe this strikes you as too "New Age", or maybe downright implausible. But stick with me a little longer.

To use a computer technology analogy, I like to think of the Elite Development Course as having three components. Master John gives you upgraded hardware. This is in the form of a celestial central nervous system. You now have the ability to run the more sophisticated, frequency identifying, internal software that he installs into your new celestial nervous system. He then establishes the equivalent of a high capacity fiber optic communication cable that directly links you with the celestial angelic kingdom. Lastly, he creates the opportunity for you to develop your own personal relationship with the Master Healing Angels. This relationship allows you to request help from the Master Healing Angels, which will or will not be granted due to the many variables we will discuss later in this book.

You, as an Elite Development Course graduate, have now been given the beginners equivalent of doing what Master John Douglas does. You can now start to "co-create" your own "Medical Miracles" by invoking and requesting help from the Master Healing Angels, who are the ones who actually do the healing and perform the miracle.

So how does this co-creation of a miracle for a given disease state actually work? Once the Elite Development Course graduate, by the art of scanning, has identified the root causative infectious agent responsible for a given "incurable" disease, then the Master Healing Angels shatter that infectious agent with a precise sonic frequency pulse analogous to the way in which an opera singer can shatter a crystal glass. We, as humans, do not have the cosmic technology to initiate the curative affect that this precise sonic frequency creates. But, luckily, we have earned the right and authority to begin to culture a relationship with the Master Healing Angels who initiate this healing upon our request.

Not all course participants wish to focus on developing the ability to heal themselves or others. They have the choice to develop these skills or not. Most course participants are more focused on their own spiritual evolution, their quest to know their Divine Nature more fully. It is a personal choice to choose one of these paths or both of them. There is no judgement from Master John as to how these abilities are used. He only asks that you take this blessing seriously to maximize the opportunities he is making available to you in this lifetime.

A description of the Elite Development Course is available on the www.masterangels.org website.

So why is the existence of, and the actual opportunity to take the Elite Development Course, so important?

From my standpoint, whether one chooses to take the course or not, is a very personal decision. The decision to attend the Elite Development Course is dictated by free time, interest and finances. But the fact that this body of knowledge is not restricted to Master John Douglas, and is transferable to ordinary folk like us, is very important from an academic and scientific standpoint.

This ability to train others satisfies the scientific requirement for reproducibility. The fact that others can verify what I am saying for themselves, by their own inner experience of scanning and invoking the Master Healing Angels, will dispel the Doubting Thomas' among us. To create an intended manifestation of healing, to kill a virus, or to positively affect a given situation in a measurable way is a deal maker from my perspective.

For me, the fact that 500 other Elite Development Course graduates, including many health professionals, have verified the reality of these claims is HUGE. It is probably the reason I am willing to risk my professional reputation to make this information available to the general public, especially when all of my professional friends have urged me to author this book under an alias.

For if I am suffering from a massive delusion regarding all that I have documented, so too, are many other medical doctors, nurses, chiropractors, naturopathic doctors, and highly successful business leaders in all walks of life.

Each of us, as graduates of one or more Elite Development Courses, have verified this knowledge on the level of our own experience. By establishing our personal relationship with the Master Healing Angels and invoking their help, many Elite Course graduates have been able to duplicate the medical miracles illustrated here and elsewhere. Our earlier story in this book, where the recent Elite Course graduate was able to request help from the Master Healing Angels in order to heal her own fungal skin lesion so soon after taking the Elite Development

Course is a typical example of how quickly this proficiency can develop.

So, a legitimate follow-up question would be: "Do I, Dr. Richard Sarnat, use these abilities in my medical practice with my patients?"

The short answer is that "no." I do not use these techniques with my patients. But that is partly because I am no longer in clinical practice actively seeing patients in an office setting.

While I do still write pharmaceutical prescriptions as medically indicated, confer with emergency rooms on the appropriateness of medical admissions, confer with specialists on the appropriateness of a given workup or treatment plan, my professional responsibilities in my current occupation are more administrative as a Medical Director and Chief Medical Officer of a managed care company. Hopefully this helps explain why my answer is "no," as to the question of my professional use of Master John's knowledge in a clinical setting.

However, the reasons go deeper than that. The description of scanning and invoking the Master Healing Angels is not within the current realm of medical science as we know it. These ideas and actions are currently within the realm of theology.

While the technical abilities and expertise of invoking the Master Healing Angels in a given situation is highly technical and predictable for graduates of the Elite Development Course, essentially, we are still talking about a form of prayer. Last I checked, Ministers, Rabbis, Pastors and all other forms of clergy

do not practice medicine, even if they are so fortunate as to trigger a medical miracle by prayer.

Given, that as a medical doctor, my recommendations will automatically be understood as coming from a scientific perspective by someone who is licensed to practice medicine, and not a theological perspective, I try to not mix the two worlds.

In the same vein, this book is best understood as my attempt to be a medical historian, thinking aloud as you and I take this journey to try to explain how all of these miraculous phenomena make scientific sense.

As such, a typical medical disclaimer is very much in order. Please keep in mind, that while it is true that I am a medical professional, the knowledge that is being presented in this book has been taught to me by The Church of the Master Angels, a diverse international congregation focused on Spiritual Development and **whose products are not intended to diagnose, treat, cure or prevent any disease or illness.** As their website states: "If you have any health concerns, we strongly **suggest consulting a qualified healthcare professional for diagnosis and treatment options.**"

The Church of the Master Angels website lists a more detailed medical disclaimer. I fully agree with the importance of this disclaimer and want to make certain that you, the reader, understand the full nature of faith-based healings.

By visiting this website, I acknowledge, understand, and have faith that references to the **concepts of healing or treatments**

on this website are describing faith-based blessings performed by God and the Master Angels and are not performed by any individual or affiliate of CMA International or the Church of the Master Angels. CMA International, the Church of the Master Angels, or any of their affiliates, speakers, or representatives do not offer medical advice. The statements and advice offered on this website have not been independently evaluated by the medical community.

The products and items on this website are not intended to diagnose, treat, cure, or prevent any disease or medical condition. **The products and items on this website, which also are discussed within this book, are not substitutes for prudent medical care offered by a licensed medical professional.**

This disclaimer begs us to answer two additional, interesting questions. What is the role of faith to the success or failure of miraculous healing? And, on what level does a miraculous healing actually occur?

Our next case study will help us answer these two questions.

11

Systemic Lupus Erythematosus (SLE) and the Future Role of Divinity in Medicine

Our patient, who we will call Sandy, is a 40-year-old, white, female who first met Master John Douglas in 2007, while she was in good health. Unfortunately, by 2009 the status of her "good health' had changed and she was diagnosed with the incurable autoimmune disease known as SLE. Believing that her disease was incurable, her physician introduced her to an SLE support group, "so she would be reality-based about her future."

Looking back to 2009 Sandy would describe her symptoms as: "Severe pain inside my bones as if my bones were frozen. My pain was at a constant nine out of ten level. I had very low energy and a constant undiagnosed flu-like syndrome with muscle aches." Formerly a professional dancer, she now required a hot bath first thing in the morning just to be able to move at all. Dancing was out of the question.

Attempting to find an alternative medical cure, she tried hyperbaric oxygen chambers, intravenous oxygen infusion, acupuncture and homeopathy. None of these alternative modalities stopped her disease progression or succeeded in offering her permanent relief.

Her symptoms continued to become progressively

worse until 2010 when she again saw Master John Douglas in Santa Barbara, California. As soon as she saw him, she reports that: "I had a complete shift in my overall well-being. I knew I would be cured." By the time she left the session, she experienced a 100% improvement in symptoms. However, Master John Douglas warned her that: "her disease would not be fully healed until he could work on a deeper level."

This turned out to be true. She experienced a slow relapse to about 20%-30% of her former symptoms. She did, however, attempt to go to every seminar he gave within the state of California, which amounted to seeing him six to eight times annually.

During this early phase of her recovery, she also reports using tourmaline detoxification foot patches daily, taking detoxification salt baths three or four times weekly and using the micronutrient mineral supplementation that was suggested by Master John Douglas.

The final and complete miraculous healing occurred when Master John released a new audio healing process called Soul Repair. Once Master John was literally able to affect a healing at the soul level, and she chose to listen to the audio of Soul Repair daily, her recovery became 100% stable, without any recurrence of symptoms. She now is able to resume all of her former activities, such as dancing.

Quite a story and one of my favorite case reports for many reasons.

Like all of the previous case studies of auto-immune diseases, Lupus always has an underlying occult infectious etiology. **In my opinion, the human physiology is**

simply too well designed and too well-engineered to attack itself erroneously, without provocation. I believe that over time, medical science will find that all diseases currently classified as "autoimmune diseases" will all be found to have an occult infectious etiology.

Master John Douglas was able to discern that Lupus is caused by a mold, coupled with a coexistent symbiotic-bacteria, which then eats the mold and the duo together deposit their toxins in any organ, such as kidney, liver or spleen. Killing the mold and the bacteria that live by ingesting the mold results in a cure.

Yet, in the early phase of her healing, before the Soul Repair audio became available, she was still suffering with the disease. While her symptoms and quality of life definitely improved, a complete and stable miraculous healing was not achieved. This gives us a glimpse into deeper Laws of Nature that govern true miraculous healing and long-term remissions.

What are these deeper laws?

When a medical doctor makes a differential diagnosis and looks at all the possible causes for a given disease, it is like peeling back an onion to reveal the many layers or natural law.

The cause of a given disease could be:

• Food born–infectious or not.

• Air born–infectious or not.

• Environmental toxicity

• Infectious vector, such as Lyme disease

• Genetic

• Epigenetic, which is triggered by the environment

- Mutagenic/cancer
- Hormonal
- Metabolic

The list goes on and on.

Any good diagnostician will consider all of these options and many more. But few, if any physicians, will consider whether the disease actually originated on the level of the soul.

This brings us back to the end of the last chapter and the need for a medical disclaimer. Clearly, once again, a discussion of a given disease being determined on the level of the soul sounds much more theological than within the realm of medical science.

And yet, what are we to do with this additional data point and the fact that a full healing in this person was not achievable until Master John was "allowed" to create the Soul Repair tool?

Does this reveal an even deeper layer of the onion, so to speak, than the nine well known conventional medical diagnostic options listed above?

I think we have to answer, "yes" to that question and dig a little deeper into what a healing on the level of the soul really means.

12

Spiritual Energy Bodies

Now that we have a case study where Master John could not perform a complete and stable miraculous healing until the healing was performed on the level of the soul, I guess we are committed to believing that the soul is real and not just a fairy tale in religious lore.

As an Elite Development Course graduate, I am happy to reveal that the soul has its own unique frequency, like everything else in nature. One of the great revelations of the ability to scan the frequency of everything in nature is to verify for oneself the actual existence of the soul, and many other such interesting scientifically/theologically debatable concepts.

Yes, I am going on record as both a scientist and an amateur theologian, that the soul exists and is just one of a number of discrete and measurable energy bodies. From a medical standpoint, even more importantly, the seat of disease, or the root cause of a chronic dysfunction, can actually exist at the level of these unseen energy bodies, these deeper, more subtle levels of our existence.

Let's go back to the interview with Master John, written by Amber Terrrell, and see what he had to say about the root causes of disease and their relationship to the existence of these subtle, spiritual bodies.

Q: *How do you see your abilities and your mission in relation to allopathic medicine, which tends to focus on symptoms rather than causes?*

John: The process of being able to scan frequencies has allowed me to find many cures and treatments for diseases that are not understood by current medical science. It allows me to see where science may be coming in from the wrong angle. Now, I love western medicine. And, I love science. **But the truth is, with all our advanced technology and learning, doctors are not always looking in the right place to properly cure a condition. From the perspective I have, it's clear that disease often doesn't start in the physical. Trauma, emotional and mental stress, false belief systems and blocks to our personal growth can be stored in the energy fields of our bodies and be impacting our ability to function at our full potential.** These blocks obstruct the vital flow of energy through our body, energy that is necessary for our health and well-being. **Over time this blockage leads to illness and depleted mental and emotional reserves. Powerful energetic healing can restore these vital flows.**

Q: *Suppose I was suffering from back pain. How would your ability to read these frequencies help me in a different way than a traditional physician might?*

John: Okay, let's say you go to your doctor with lower back pain, mild lower back pain, and you are prescribed muscle relaxants, or pain killers, which brings some temporary relief. But if you had the ability to scan the frequencies that are there in your lower back, you may be able to determine what is really going on. Is there a small, localized infections in your kidney ducts causing inflammation? Are there bacteria? Are your kidney ducts swollen to a degree and burning? Is the pain coming from there? Usually, something like that is going on with many types of back pain.

Q: *And you can actually see this?*

John: Yes, I can see it and identify it. That's what I have in the way of this frequency-tuning tool, which is far more valuable than clairvoyance. A probe of my consciousness can enter any point in time and space and I can, by elimination, tune to any frequency I desire to identify energy or matter and really determine what's happening with your back pain, what its ultimate cause could be. Is it something karmic? Is it something just as a result of clumsiness? Is it something caused by free will or choice? **If you could really see what was causing the problem, you could get rid of it and not have to cover up the symptoms with medicine.**

Q: *Symptom-suppressing drugs are very lucrative in this country. We don't have the socialized medicine system like you have in Australia.*

John: The fact that we have this kind of system recently helped to document the recovery of one of my clients. This lady had been diagnosed with an autoimmune disorder Multiple Sclerosis (MS) that was deteriorating her nerves. She was getting fortnightly interferon injections from the hospital. Now, because of our type of medical system, it doesn't cost $3000 every time you get a CAT scan. It's free. So, if you're receiving some kind of ongoing treatment, you will be scanned every time you come in just to make sure you really need it. And so, when I started working with this lady, she was getting scanned twice a month. **When I looked at her, I could see that the myelin sheath, the insulating covering around nerves, was being eaten away by microorganisms and that they were excreting a waste product that was inflaming her nerves. All this was making her begin to lose vision and lose balance. So, I killed the microorganisms with an impulse of consciousness and cleared out her body of the toxins by neutralizing their frequency.** When she went back for her next interferon appointment a week and half later, they scanned her brain and did not see the inflammation. They weren›t sure what was going on but decided not to give her the injection that day. I got a joyful email from her sister: "They've delayed her injections!" **Two weeks later, at her next appointment, the scan did not show the condition to be present at all and they took her off the program altogether. And that's not a miracle. It's just finding something medical science hasn't found yet. Because I can accurately scan the body.**

Q: *That story would've been hard to believe a few months ago. But I happen to know someone who was suffering from Lyme Disease and was recently cured by you. Some would call that almost miraculous, because*

I don't think traditional medicine has a cure for Lyme, do they?

John: I know it seems miraculous, but it's just working with the Laws of Nature. Lyme disease is an infection from a microorganism. **How do we kill microorganisms spiritually? Well, we transmit a frequency within divine prana, a frequency that is the exact frequency of the organism. And that will electrocute the organism and eliminate it.** The situation with Lyme disease is that none of the antibiotics that doctors throw at it will work. The reason for that is because these antibiotics are carried in the bloodstream and the parasites that cause Lyme, the Borrelia bacteria, set up housekeeping in the bloodless cavities of the brain. So, it will of course not be affected by any medicine you put into the blood stream. I am able to find these parasites, by identifying their frequency and then by using a sonic pulse from consciousness destroy the organism, then recovery is a matter of cleaning out the mess left behind by the waste material of the parasites.

Q: *What about these Angelic Beings? You said that when you were young, you established a connection with some very powerful beings who helped you to develop your abilities and understand how to use them. Can you speak about this connection?*

John: Yes. This connection is the other part, the more important part, of the tool-set that allows me to do what I do. For example, killing a microorganism is something that relieves somebody's suffering. It sounds very powerful and very complicated but it's actually quite easy. It is what is working through me that gives me the right and allows me to do this. In my early twenties, I was given this direct telepathic link to some very high Angelic Beings who had an agenda for mankind. They had a dharmic purpose themselves to accelerate this path of human evolution at this particular time.

Q: *What about the energy bodies, the spiritual bodies? You implied earlier that the healing someone needs is often more than just physical.*

John: Great question. As you probably know, the physical body contains a lot of intricate systems, complicated organs and connections, and many complex chemical reactions. But I'll tell you, the spiritual bodies are just as complex. This very complicated spiritual body, the pranic body, the subtle body, the reflection of the physical body, which is unseen by many people, is just as complicated, if not more complicated than the physical body in all its functions and processes. The spiritual bodies are perfect in form, and they are very, very intensely powered by divine prana.

Q: *What do you mean by divine prana? How does it relate to imbalances in the physical body?*

John: There is a flow of prana, divine life force, that flows through the spiritual anatomy. There are meridians. These are channels that carry the prana into your body, into your senses and into your spiritual bodies. These channels are the freeways of the spiritual anatomy. And we all know what happens when the freeways get clogged up.

Q. *So, when this pranic freeway is clogged, you have a sort of road rage?*

John: The analogy isn't far off. This pranic flow can get constricted by a number of things: radiation, computers, cell phones, toxins, pesticides, medicine, recreational drugs, your emotional stress, you partner's emotional stress. All of these things can limit the pranic flow in our bodies. **And so, these bio-electric fields of the body, what some call the aura, or the light fields, these can get dirty, clogged, constricted and that can often be the precursor of illness in one form or another.** So, we have created some healing processes that are listened to which access certain processes to help you protect these bio-electric fields and keep them clean and clear. The Spirit Repair audio process, for example, has over 5,000 processes of healing and clearing that are being performed on you every nine minutes.

This sequence of the interview with Master John Douglas has a lot of esoteric concepts to digest, I admit.

1. That trauma and emotional stress can be stored in these subtler energy bodies, resulting in a blockage of pranic energy flow, or "chi", as a Doctor of Traditional Chinese Medicine would call it.

2. That failure to clear these subtle energy bodies of previous trauma can be the seed of illness which will be manifested in the physical body later.

3. That powerful energetic healings can restore the vital pranic flow, or chi, and relieve this blockage of energy, curing the patient.

4. That Multiple Sclerosis (MS), like our other case studies

of autoimmune disease, is also caused by an unknown microorganism causing inflammation of the myelin sheath and that killing the microorganism is able to quickly reverse the neurological damage seen on an MRI.

5. That listening to the audio health tools of Master John can help protect these subtle energy fields and keep them clean and clear.

While I know you need more time to digest all of these new concepts, unfortunately, there are even more layers of the onion that still need to be peeled back.

No rest for the weary on this adventure. Welcome to my world.

Let's look at another miraculous healing that illuminates the role of "worthiness", as yet another variable to help us understand why some people are blessed with a medical miracle and others not.

13

A Spontaneous Public Healing of
Chronic Trigeminal Neuralgia

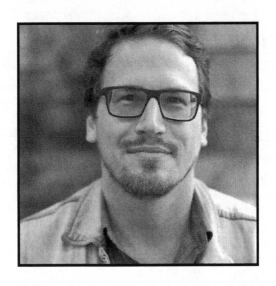

This testimonial and case study are unique in many ways. First off, the healing took place in front of 120 people at a Master John Douglas beginning-level instructional and knowledge event. This level event, by design, is tailored for people who are typically first-timers and relatively new to Master John's knowledge being presented. These beginning-level instructional events are also not intended to be a display of public healing.

As the healing of any illness is a private matter, typically Master John invokes the help of the Master

Healing Angels to evoke a healing within the privacy of a personal 5-minute session behind closed doors.

However, there is one opportunity for public healing to occur at what is referred to as a C-level event. These rare events are highly cherished by the Elite Development Course graduates. These C-level events are the only opportunity for Elite Development Course graduates to follow the decision tree and frequencies revealed by Master John as he spontaneously, without prior information, attempts to heal individuals in front of a large public audience and worldwide telephonic audience. A perusal of the www.masterangels.org website will provide a clear description of how the different public events are organized.

In the ten years that I have watched and listened to Master John Douglas at these various events, I have never seen him spontaneously do an unscheduled public healing at an entry level event. So those of us who have been around for a while, knew immediately that something unusual was happening at this event.

This medical miracle involves a 40-year-old named Mike who suffered through what he describes as, "debilitating oral surgery" at age three to correct the trauma he experienced when he was kicked in the face by a horse. Immediately after being kicked in the face, he lost all four of his front baby teeth and ultimately only two of his four adult teeth survived.

From the ages of 11 through 18 he had temporary posts placed and underwent many surgeries, which culminated in severe bone and tissue loss. All attempts at bone grafting ultimately failed. Between the ages of 36 to 38, he underwent 6 major procedures in an attempt to achieve success using modern implants.

Unfortunately, subsequent to these many surgeries, he began to permanently have both a burning and tingling sensation in his face that became progressively worse.

At this juncture, Mike saw a Neurologist who made the diagnosis of Trigeminal Neuralgia. The Neurologist attempted to control the pain with anticonvulsant medication, but the side effects were unbearable. Desperate to have some improvement, all the implants were removed. He was left with major bone loss, gum recession and scarring.

He sought out the help of a pain specialist and at one point was taking up to eight Vicodin, a synthetic opioid, daily without finding relief. He then looked to the alternative medicine world and luckily found an Elite Development Course graduate whom he credits with "helping him immensely." Mike also credits this Naturopathic physician with significantly helping him during this period and relates that together they surmised that his Trigeminal Neuralgia might actually be virally induced.

While he still felt that he had to use whiskey and cannabis at times to survive hour to hour, slowly, by listening to the recommended Master John Douglas audio Health Repair tools, he began to experience some relief.

Prior to the Master John event in San Diego, Mike remembers that on a daily basis he listened to the various health audio Repair tools of: Karmic Repair, Soul Repair, and Psychology Repair. He also listened to Subconscious Repair once a week as is recommended.

Mike remembers being very nervous the night before the Master John Douglas seminar. He was concerned as to whether or not he was "worthy of receiving a cure." He relates that despite this existential musing: "I eventually reached a place of faith and peace that I would get what I needed at the event."

This is quite a leap of faith, as he described his pain at the time as being an eight out of ten, twenty-four hours per day. In retrospect, he believes that he was functioning at about 25% of normality during the three years before attending this Master John Douglas seminar.

Mike attended this entry-level instructional and knowledge event with his wife, his first time ever seeing Master John live or even on video. He describes his wife as a "go-getter." She immediately made sure that they had seats in the middle of the front row.

At this event, Chris Hartnett, who typically introduces Master John, spontaneously asked members of the audience to stand up and shout out for which disease they had received a miracle cure.

Confused by everyone standing up and shouting out the disease they formerly had, Mike, likewise, stood up and yelled out "Trigeminal Neuralgia."

Mike remembers that after he shouted out "Trigeminal Neuralgia" that the eyes of Master John Douglas locked on to his and he immediately "felt a break in my consciousness, as if I were riding a roller-coaster and momentarily blacked out. I remember seeing Master

John move his hands around and then instantly my pain decreased from a ten out of ten to a five out of ten."

Mike also remembers that once the initial decrease in pain occurred, that Master John asked all the Elite Development Course graduates to scan his pain receptors. Master John told the Elite Course Graduates that they would find toxins in his pain receptors that had to be cleared before the pain level would further decrease and approach zero.

Sure enough, Mike reports, that "once everyone focused on my pain receptors, my pain further diminished to a one out of ten, and it has remained so since that day, even though I never had a personal session with Master John following the group event."

Mike describes his life prior to meeting Master John Douglas as: "A nightmare. I went from being an easy-going, mellow guy, to living in an anxious, existential terror, which gave me a fight or flight response which was easily triggered at any moment."

He reports that: "The medications that I was given by my alternative medical doctor helped some. But, I was not really able to rise above the pain on a consistent basis. All of that is 100% gone now. That hyper-vigilance of fight or flight is in my past."

Of interest is that Mike describes himself as a skeptic in general. "Five years ago, I would have thought this was all bullshit. Now my life has changed from night to day."

Mike's social history is significant for the fact that his father was a physician in general medical practice. In retrospect, he believes he probably was over-prescribed with antibiotics as a child. He believes that this might have been a contributing factor to his harboring of a chronic virus.

I remember Mike's case study very clearly, as I attended the San Diego C-event remotely by telephone. I was also scanning him—first for the evidence of the virus within his facial nerve and then for the evidence of the toxins blocking full recovery of his pain receptors back to normal.

These public healings are great teaching moments for the Elite Development Course graduates and mimic what grand rounds accomplish for medical students and residents. Of course, the big difference is that the healing is accomplished by invoking the Master Healing Angels, not by any conventional medical strategy.

Luckily, while preparing to write this book, I was able to question Master John about this most unusual healing. He related the following memories:

"During the introduction, I could see that an individual in the front row was in great discomfort. I interrupted the current speaker, Chris Hartnett, to verify that he was in pain. When I asked where the pain was located, the individual said it was in his facial nerve. I was then easily able to find an unidentified virus within the facial nerve which was surrounded by inflammation. That same virus frequency was present in his intestines. I proceeded to kill the virus which created immediate relief from an eight out of ten to a two out of ten within thirty seconds. He returned the next day feeling even better.

As you know, it is not a common practice to heal anyone at the beginning of the seminar. **So, it must**

be noted that he had used our development Repair tools for three months, listening to Karmic Repair daily prior to attending the seminar. This elevated his worthiness. This happened in front of 120 people in the audience, completely unscripted and spontaneously."

Master John's comments are interesting for a number of reasons.

1. When a person is worthy to receive a special healing, how intricately the Laws of Nature organize to make that healing happen. It is most unusual for someone who has never seen Master John previously to sit in the front row, as that area is usually reserved for the Elite Course graduates.

2. Chris Hartnett, during his introduction of Master John, requested that participants in the audience stand up and shout out their miracle, which created the opportunity for this healing to occur the way it did.

3. This individual created his own worthiness by utilizing the audio Health Repair tools in preparation, prior to the actual event. This prior usage of the audio Repair tools to increase one's worthiness has been a recurrent theme seen in many of the more dramatic healings, such as the cases involving Chronic Lyme disease and Sarcoidosis.

4. The discrepancy between the subject's impression of his pain decrease versus Master John's scan of his actual pain receptors is not unusual. Individuals have subconscious barriers to appreciating the improving pain levels and often, as in this case, have residual toxins at the level of the pain

receptors that require an energetic clearing.

5. Finally, it is always important to check the intestines for the same toxins or infectious life forms that are seen at the primary disease site, which, in this case, was the facial nerve. This ties the original entry point of the infection to the gastrointestinal tract and probable tainted food ingestion. This also helps illuminate the subject's parallel development of mental health issues, as toxins in the intestines are a sign of "leaky gut syndrome." Often these same toxins travel up to the brain creating secondary behavioral health issues, such as triggering his fight or flight response.

So, in answer to the question: "Why do some people receive a miracle and not others?" We can now count an individual's worthiness as another one of the key variables.

Are there other variables? Undoubtedly so. This now brings us to an even more confusing discussion as to the definition and role of karma in both disease and in the manifestation of a miracle.

14

The Role of Karma

Let's go to Wikipedia and educate ourselves about the definition of karma.

Karma (car-ma) is a word meaning the result of a person's actions, as well as the actions themselves. **It is a term about the cycle of cause and effect.** According to the theory of karma, what happens to a person, happens because they caused it with their actions. It is an important part of many religions such as Hinduism and Buddhism.

The theory of karma can be thought to be an extension to Newton's third law of action and reaction where every action of any kind including words, thoughts, feelings, the totality of our existence, will eventually have a reaction, namely, the same type of energy coming back to the one that caused it.

In terms of spiritual development, karma is about all that a person has done, is doing and will do. Karma is not about punishment or reward. It makes a person responsible for his or her own life, and how he or she treats other people. Karma means action and reaction: if we show goodness, we will reap goodness.

Karma is the universal principle of cause and effect. Our actions, both good and bad, come back to us, helping us to learn life's lessons and become better people.

In religions that include reincarnation, our past life karma creates our present and future life situations.

Karma is basically energy. One person throws out energy through their thoughts, words and actions. It comes back, in time, through other people. Karma is the best teacher. It forces people to face the consequences of their own actions and thus improve and refine their behavior or suffer if they do not. Even harsh karma, when faced in wisdom, can be the greatest spark for spiritual growth.

The process of action and reaction on all levels, physical, mental and spiritual, is karma. One must pay attention to thoughts, because thought can make karmas, both good, bad and mixed.

Some examples.

"I say kind words to you and you feel peaceful and happy. I say harsh words to you and you become ruffled and upset. The kindness and the harshness will return to me, through others, at a later time. Finally, what I give is what I get back."

"An architect thinks creative, productive thoughts while drawing plans for a new building. But were he to think destructive, unproductive thoughts, he would soon not be able to accomplish any kind of positive task even if he desired to do so."

According to the definitions and concepts above, the manifestation of an illness must be due to some karma in this life, or from karma which we have brought with us from a past life.

Another way to think about this is the concept of

"imbalance" or living out of tune with Natural Law. In Traditional Chinese medicine, or in Indian Ayurvedic medicine, it is this "imbalance" or dis-ease which is seen diagnostically by various physical signs. Our tongue is the wrong color or has a coating. We have an abnormal pulse.

In conventional western medicine, we too recognize signs of imbalance. An abnormal heart rhythm or the presence of jaundice are two examples of well-known signs of imbalance within conventional medical diagnoses. But in conventional medicine, we do not have a holistic view of health similar to the more ancient, traditional systems of medicine.

Similar to our discussion about the soul, we now find ourselves again treading the murky waters of spiritual energy bodies, which are essentially unknown to conventional medical science.

Let's think back to what Master John said about how various energies can be stuck in the spiritual bodies from previous events and that no true healing can occur until those energies are resolved.

"The process of being able to scan frequencies has allowed me to find many cures and treatments for diseases that are not understood by medical science, and also to see where science may be coming in from the wrong angle. Now, I love western medicine, and I love science. But the truth is, with all our advanced technology and learning, **doctors are not always looking in the right place to properly cure a condition**. From the perspective I have, it's clear that disease often doesn't start in the physical. **Trauma, emotional and mental**

stress, false belief systems and blocks to our personal growth can be stored in the energy fields of our bodies and be impacting our ability to function at our full potential. These blocks obstruct the vital flow of energy through our body and systems, energy that is necessary for our health and well-being. **Over time this blockage leads to illness and depleted mental and emotional reserves. Powerful energetic healing can restore these vital flows."**

It is no accident that many of his audio Health Repair tools work on the level of the spiritual energy bodies as well as the level of the soul. This is evident in the very names of these Repair tools: Soul Repair, Soul Elevation, Karmic Repair and Spirit Repair.

This is also why the Church of the Master Angels website has two different blessings available at the top of the homepage. When you click on the "remote healings" tab, you can order a "Silent Faith Remote" blessing which is like a rifle shot, where you can describe the exact nature of your illness and the Master Angels will attend to it specifically. Or, you can order a "Karmic Mitigation" blessing which works on a much deeper layer to attempt to rebalance whatever is out of balance with the Laws of Nature and with past karma.

In my experience, after watching many people go through the healing process, it seems that these two blessings are best used in tandem for any major disease manifestation. This is especially true for stubborn chronic diseases, where the disease seems to have deep roots at some level of our energy bodies. Master John has recently given us a basic formula to resolve the most stubborn and deep-seated chronic illnesses:

> *Listen to Soul Repair and Karmic Repair daily; Repeat both a Silent Faith Remote blessing and a Karmic Mitigation blessing every three weeks until the situation is satisfactorily resolved.*

Why is this the prescribed formula for the resolution of chronic disease? While I have never heard Master John specifically discuss the reasons behind these exact instructions, I have my own theory, which is the following: It is important that we take some personal responsibility for being part of our own solution, hence the requirement of three weeks of active participation using the Repair tools before requesting either of the remote faith healings on the website. So, while we lay the groundwork by doing three weeks of Repair tools, our inability to affect the deeper levels of our own personal karma, which is where the imbalance that creates the disease is stored, requires the intervention of the Master Healing Angels to mitigate on our behalf.

To look at it from a different perspective, this formula seems to be designed to help us elevate our worthiness by our own actions, as well as being more deserving to ask and receive the help we request.

It is also my experience that we all underestimate the amount of past karma that has been accumulated and how it directly and indirectly affects everything in our daily lives. This is why a key component of the Elite Development Course is character development: how to use one's new found scanning abilities to discern right from wrong action, action that creates positive karma versus action that creates negative karma.

Each type of karma, positive versus negative, emits a different frequency which can be known. So, scanning becomes a very useful tool to end the cycle of "less than optimal behavior" as the Elite Course Graduate attempts to improve his or her character.

Master John is famous for saying that: "Someone can meditate for forty years and still be so obnoxious that no one wants to be their friend." Meditation alone, Yoga alone, Tai Chi alone—none of these practices give us the ability to discern right action, which creates positive karma, from wrong action that creates negative karma.

This is not a criticism of these wonderful spiritual and health practices, which have stood the test of time over many millennia. Rather, it is just to point out the deeper layers of discernment that are available to graduates of the Elite Development Course, once their scanning faculties have been accurately established.

So, let's talk about how scanning is developed in a little more detail.

15

The Art of Scanning to Cultivate Discernment

We started our discussions early in the book by acknowledging that both Einstein and Tesla believed that the organization of the universe could be best understood by the study of frequencies.

> *"Everything is energy and that's all there is. Match the frequency of the reality you want, and you cannot help but get that reality. It can be no other way. This is not philosophy, this is physics."* Albert Einstein

> *"Future medicine will be the medicine of frequencies."* Albert Einstein

> *"If you want to find the secrets of the universe, think in terms of energy, frequency and vibration."* Nikola Tesla

While I certainly agree with our two eminent scientists as to their assessment of the structure of the universe, how can we make sense on a practical day-to day basis of the infinite range of frequencies to be analyzed? And, how does this apply specifically to medical science?

My favorite Master John Douglas quote helps to point us in the right direction: *"Everything in the universe is separated by frequency and unified by consciousness."*

To say it another way, it is only through the study of consciousness that we will be able to understand how the universe functions at its deepest levels, creating and recreating itself again and again, by using an infinite number of sound frequencies.

Master John Douglas teaches his Elite Development students a mental practice that he calls scanning. At times, it is also referred to as divining. Scanning is a consciousness-based technique. This means that it is done within the mind of the scanner. An outside observer is not able to see what is happening inside of the mind of the scanner. They can only see the results. This is similar to someone doing a math problem in their head. You can't see how their mind is determining how to add two to five until they verbally tell you that the correct answer is seven.

Scanning is a gift given to the student by Master John during the Elite Development Course. Master John upgrades the student on the level of their physiology, then gives them a "software download" to enable the scanning ability. Like any skill set, the student's accuracy develops over time and with practice.

Quantum Physics tells us that all particles of matter emit light and sound in a spectrum of infinite frequencies. The art of scanning, experienced by the student on the level of the deep inner mind, enables the student to sense the frequency of any particular particle of matter.

The "hardware upgrade" that Master John empowers in the Elite student stimulates the pineal gland and turns it into a very refined central processing unit, similar to a high-powered computer server. Master John then utilizes the upgraded palm chakras, which are also glands and function as energy sensors in the hands of the body, as an output device. The software download directs the output devices, the palm chakras, to measure the requested frequency and report the results in a more physical form. This is analogous to how a computer directs a printer, an output device that is connected to it, to report the results of what it has just processed. Simultaneously, on the level of one's inner consciousness, the answer to the question that was posed before the scan comes to the mind of the Elite student, just like a computer search result comes to the screen of the computer. The student now has the result of their inquiry reported to them in two forms. They can feel the result in their hands and know the result in their mind.

If we go deeper into the biological hardware upgrade that Master John installs in the Elite Development Course students, we can look at what he calls the "scanning matrix." This is an internal, internet-like biological network.

The first component of the matrix is the pineal gland which has multi-pointed and multi-dimensional capabilities. This gland is like an internal, biological computer processor that is connected to the infinite possibilities and infinite correlation that exists on the subtlest quantum mechanical levels of the whole universe. The Elite Development Course unlocks this biological super computer capability within the pineal gland. The course participant can now shed the human illusion of the linear time-space continuum and begin to live in a reality which is an unbounded field of infinite possibilities.

The palm chakras are the second major component of the matrix. They are biological glands that act as energy sensors. In the sciences of Indian Ayurveda and Chinese Traditional medicine, these energy sensors are known as marma points and acupuncture points. These energy centers in the palms are another component of the biological matrix upgraded by Master John in the Elite Development Course student.

While Master John Douglas has a distinct advantage over the Elite Development Course graduates due to his ability to utilize 19 clairvoyant senses, he is always quick to point out that all of his discoveries could have been made by scanning alone. Yes, he certainly can "see" directly any unseen disease in the body that we, as graduates, must find by using our scanning abilities and by discerning between various frequencies. But the lesson is well-taken.

I mentioned before that another gift that Master John gives his Elite students is a cosmic "legal contract" with those beings in the universe who are experts in human physiology. They are experts because they were given the assignment by the Creator to actually engineer and help manufacture the first human bodies. Just like a grad student who is working on their doctorate degree is assigned a Faculty advisor, each new Elite student is assigned a Master Healing Angel to assist them in learning how to scan. Eventually, with practice, practice and more practice scanning by the Elite student, the Master Healing Angels "take off the training wheels" and the Elite student is fully able to scan accurately on his or her own.

So, what are the current limits of this knowledge? How far can this technology go in creating future medical miracles? Our next two medical miracles will help to answer these questions.

16

What are the Limits of Healing?

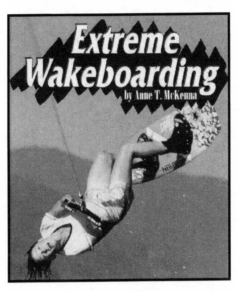

Case Study One: Delayed Onset Prosthetic Joint Infection (PJI), Successfully Treated for Eight Months Without the use of Surgery or Antibiotics.

Meet my close friend, Dana who is a 46-year-old retired professional athlete. She is an X-Games World Champion and Hall of Fame wakeboarder. In 1999 and 2001, she suffered through two major left knee ACL reconstructions. On January 31, 2017, having essentially no meniscus, cartilage or functional ACL, she took the extraordinary measure of having a total knee replacement at age 43. The good news is that four months after her original surgery, life was good, and her recovery was on schedule as expected.

The bad news is that suddenly on May 7, 2017, for no apparent reason, the knee began to have increased swelling, redness, pain and heat. Her symptoms waxed and waned for ten days. Being an Elite Graduate myself, I attempted to invoke the Master Healing Angels to affect a miracle cure.

But, as we have discussed, at this time on our planet there are limits to what miracles can accomplish. So, after ten days of attempting to perform a miracle, I "waved the white flag" and presented Dana to the local emergency room with a pain scale of ten out of ten. The next day, May 12, 2017, at a university-affiliated emergency room where her Orthopedists were on staff, she had the fluid on her knee aspirated and she was sent home to await the cell counts and fluid analysis which would determine her surgeon's next steps.

At about 9 pm that same night, Dana received a call regarding her lab reports. Her tests indicated a severe bacterial infection of her artificial left knee prosthesis. The Orthopedic surgeon on call recommended immediate admission to the hospital so that emergency surgery could take place the next morning. She was told that the surgery most likely would involve removal of the left knee implant, insertion of an antibiotic poly-methyl methacrylate spacer and ongoing intravenous antibiotic therapy for approximately eight weeks.

Needless to say, this was not good news, as there is both a significant risk of amputation, and even death, secondary to a confirmed bacterial prosthetic joint infection.

So, while Dana was in tears, I began to drive her to the university emergency room for a preplanned admission in preparation for emergency surgery the next morning. Luckily, while driving to the hospital, I was able to reach Master John Douglas by telephone.

Pulling the car off of the road at a nearby gas station, I proceeded to explain Dana's situation and the fact that I was unable to successfully invoke a miraculous cure despite my repeated efforts to do so. I simply could not identify the infecting agent, which I knew both intuitively, and by medical training, had to be present in her knee joint.

I, as an Elite Development Course graduate of many years now, had already initiated many miraculous healings by requesting help from those who actually do the healing, the Master Healing Angels. However, in all of those cases, I had first successfully identified the frequency of a specific bacteria or virus which proved to be the root cause of the given disease. In Dana's case, I was unable to locate the root cause of her infection. I simply could not "hear the song emanating from that life form."

Master John remotely looked into Dana's body and told me that Dana was infected by an organism unknown to conventional medicine. This organism had the frequency of what he calls a "pharmaceutical negative animal." Unfortunately, this frequency was, up to this point, unknown to me. I had never heard its song before through my scanning efforts. It was not in my pineal glands supercomputer database yet. This explains why I could not find it as I was looking and listening for the typical strep or staph bacterial infections that are found with most prosthetic joint infections.

As soon as I was given the name of the frequency by Master John, I was easily able to locate its existence and watch its frequency signal fade away as Master John invoked the Master Healing Angels to kill the infectious entities within Dana's body, by using a sonic frequency which would shatter their integrity. I could follow the decreasing trend of inflammation as time passed after Master John's intervention. This is the beauty of being able to scan. The real-time tracking through the technology of scanning of the unseen root causes that create one disease manifestation or another.

Now we came to a moment of truth for Dana. This was not my knee and not my life on the line. **Remember, I am not giving her medical advice, from the position of a physician discussing the standard of care for a given situation. I am just a close friend who is lucky enough to be able to witness a miracle in action as it unfolds before me.**

I turned to Dana and told her what Master John had said and what the Master Healing Angels had accomplished. I told her: "Yes, I was able to witness this and verify for myself the eradication of the infectious agent. But I reminded her that this was a life and death situation and that only she could make the decision about what to do next."

The choice was binary. I asked: "Do you have enough

faith in Master John and myself to risk your life, turn around and go home, and hope you are alive when you awake in the morning? Or, do you want me to keep driving to the emergency room and proceed with surgery tomorrow morning, as is the standard of care for this disease process?"

In one of the greatest leaps of faith I have ever witnessed, Dana responded that, her faith in Master John and my ability to accurately scan what took place were good enough for her and that we should turnaround and head back home.

More than just a leap of faith, this was also an act of great courage by Dana. Remember, though, that we are dealing with an X-game world champion who has spent her life defying the odds with crazy aerial stunts twenty feet up in the air that no sane person, like me, would even consider yet alone attempt. In my defense, I am burdened by having gone to medical school and by knowing the natural history of prosthetic joint infections. Dana was being very innocent in her unwavering faith in the power of Master John Douglas to perform miracles.

Was this faith illogical, given her past experiences with Master John?

No, not in the least illogical.

After all, she had been to many public seminars and even two Elite Development Courses by this time. She had met hundreds of people who had given testimonials as to their own miraculous healings.

But knowing all of the mysteries revealed in the Elite Development Course and hearing other people's testimonies about their miraculous healings is still very different from needing your own miracle to survive. Furthermore, when one has an illness as severe as this, the accuracy of scanning for oneself is suspect and so Dana had no choice but to take a leap of faith (or not).

Truth be told, while I totally agreed with her decision and was very proud of her on one level, a small medically-trained part of my brain was quite scared for her. Was she going to be septic or even worse when I poked her the next morning to check on the temperature of her skin and to make sure she was still with us?

Luckily the story trends happily. Upon waking the next morning, 90% of the pain, redness, swelling and heat that had been present in the left knee the night before had now dissipated. It was a totally unanticipated and unexplainable event from the paradigm of conventional medicine.

Was this radical improvement just a placebo effect? Or, due to a total misdiagnosis of her situation? Possibly, but highly unlikely given the severity of the cell counts seen in her aspirated left knee effusion.

Ten days after her knee had been aspirated in the emergency room and Master John Douglas' healing, instead of the predicted nonsurgical course involving increasing pain and possible sepsis, Dana's knee continued to be markedly less swollen, less hot, less painful and more mobile. Her endurance and energy now had returned to activity levels similar to before the onset of this delayed late stage infection.

In my opinion, this resolution of severe symptomatology

represents a "miracle", as it is totally unexplained by the natural course of events predicted by our conventional pathophysiological medical model. This was a surgical emergency according to conventional medicine and only a miracle could explain Dana's ability to now thrive without the use of antibiotics or surgery.

However, as is suggested by the published scientific literature on the natural history of prosthetic joint infections, this infection is difficult to eradicate. It is well-known that the inflammatory response to the infectious agents will create a biofilm, a specific type of scar tissue, that harbors the infection and makes all nonsurgical options predictably fail to achieve a cure. Would this hold true for miraculous healings as well? Unfortunately, we will see that the answer to this question is YES.

With the existence of a biofilm now most likely, the knee continued to "smolder" over a four-month course, requiring multiple Silent Faith Remote energetic healing sessions by the Master Healing Angels. Reinfections occurred with the "pharmaceutical negative animal", our original infectious agent, as well as with a variety of opportunistic staph bacteria.

I particularly remember one dramatic episode that occurred while Dana was at an Elite Development Course in North Carolina. Master John again energetically killed off all the infectious agents by invoking the Master Healing Angels. The subsequent detoxification process was so extreme that Dana had a total body rash. This rash resulted in a near complete sloughing off of her epidermis, leaving her with flaky lizard like skin, resembling severe burns. In addition, drops of grossly dark red blood started draining from her navel. This was especially odd, as Dana had no previous umbilical surgery or laparoscopy to explain this phenomenon.

After this episode, once again Dana's course trended positively. Following Master John's "killing off" of the infectious burden and the major detoxification event described above, she then remained stable without increasing signs of reinfection for two months. She was able to resume such activities as bike riding up to ten miles at a time, enjoying her paddle board and maintaining a generally high energy level.

Unfortunately, by the fall of 2017, it was clear to me clinically that the infection had not been eradicated 100%. So, she pursued a further standard conventional medical workup. After a series of culture negative knee aspirations using routine microbiology plating and cultures, Dana went on to have a polymerase chain reaction (PCR) study. PCR identifies any past or current DNA in the tissues. In this case, it identified a staphylococcus aureus. Staphylococcus is a commonly diagnosed bacteria which is often the cause of late stage surgical infections.

It is a cautionary tale that miraculous healings and medical remission can occur for a specified period of time, and yet only delay the necessity for more conventional treatment, such as in this case. Removal of the infected implant and the insertion of an antibiotic spacer was still required, as well as ten weeks of antibiotic intravenous infusion through a pic line.

Not only was this treatment regimen required thirteen

months after the original surgery but the second antibiotic filled spacer also became infected. So, for a second time, the knee spacer was removed and replaced with a new spacer and the same pic line was utilized for a second ten-week intravenous antibiotic course of treatment.

Finally, on February 19, 2019, now over two years after the original total knee replacement, Dana underwent a second total knee replacement with a much more complex prosthesis involving the placement of metal rods into the shaft of the bone itself.

As of the writing of this book, Dana is clinically improving on a daily basis. She is now seven months into an eighteen-month healing process where her bone marrow will regrow new bone tissue to properly anchor the metal rods. Our hope is that eleven months from now, Dana will once again be able to resume a very active and athletic life–although without risking "big air" as the X-Gamers would say.

On to our final case report, which again illustrates a medical miracle albeit within certain limits. I think we will find that understanding the limits of miraculous manifestations that are allowed at this time, reveals how nature is designed and provides yet another layer of truth for us to assimilate.

Case Study Two: Chronic Lymphocytic Leukemia

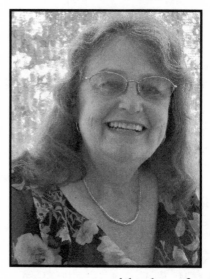

Meet Dolly, a seventy-year old white female who was first diagnosed with leukemia by finding unanticipated abnormalities on her routine blood work on July 10, 2015. She was having no clinical symptoms when she went to her appointment with her primary care doctor for a routine annual checkup and blood work. At that time, her white blood cells were mildly elevated and her platelets were slightly low.

She was immediately referred to an Oncologist who held off on using any conventional medical treatment but continued to follow her status with serial blood analysis every two or three months. During this period of time, Dolly self-treated, taking multiple herbs from a local Naturopathic physician. She observed a very restrictive diet with no sugar, gluten or dairy. However, despite her attempts at natural healing, her white blood cell counts rapidly rose over a short period of time.

In 2017, her Oncologist warned her that she had a life expectancy of three years even with standard conventional treatment. She had an increased risk factor known as a chromosome deletion of Tp53, which sits on the #17 gene.

Dolly sought out a second opinion at Duke Medical Center and conventional medical treatment was initiated as an inpatient on October 16, 2017. At this juncture, her white blood cell count was very elevated and, in short, she had the classic picture of Chronic Lymphocytic Leukemia.

By December 26, 2017, she was told that her spleen measured two times normal and it most likely would need to be surgically removed. She deferred on the immediate surgical removal of her spleen in order to see Master John Douglas at a seminar being held on June 2, 2018.

After her session with Master John on June 2, 2018, approximately two months later she had a CAT scan from the skull base to the mid thighs on August 15, 2018. This scan read as completely normal with no aggressive lesions and no abnormal activity. Her white blood cell counts also dropped to normal. This patient remains alive and active as of October 2019.

For those with a medical bent, her repeat bone marrow on June 5, 2019 showed a 5% residual CLL involvement in a 50% cellular bone marrow. No circulating blasts or abnormal lymphocytes were noted. No granulomas or metastatic tumor deposits were identified.

Were the improvements in her blood work and scans purely due to the cumulative effect of her ongoing chemotherapy? Or, was Master John Douglas responsible for the sudden positive reversal in her signs and symptoms after she initially saw him?

We will never know the answer to that question for sure. Master John often says that: "The combination of conventional chemotherapy and Angelic Reformation work hand in hand. There is a big difference between chemotherapy used alone and chemotherapy directed by Divine intention."

Of interest academically, is that following her healing performed by Master John Douglas on June 2, 2018, all the clinical signs of her CLL improved–the reduction of her splenomegaly, the normalization of her PET/CT scans and the normalization of her blood work and bone marrow. Almost everything abnormal in her labs has now returned to normal.

There is, however, one exceptional lab result which has remained abnormal. Her genetic deletion and shortened telomeres, which puts her at risk for a worse prognosis, remains the same. In other words, there was no regrowth of additional length to her telomeres to correct her mutagenic deletion on a genetic level.

The failure of her telomeres to repair and regrow is further evidence of the fact, as Master John Douglas has repeatedly told us at the Elite Development Courses, as well as stating publicly: "Not everything can be healed at this juncture in time. As the collective consciousness of the world continues to improve, then additional breakthroughs in healing will be allowed to manifest. We have not been given permission to completely cure diabetes, hypertension, genetic diseases and all forms of cancer. Nor are we allowed to reverse the central nervous system damage already incurred in many neurologic diseases and dementias. However, someday we will just be able to grow a new arm."

The optimism and certainty of this statement may seem unrealistic or delusional to the general public who have not had the good fortune to work closely with Master John and observe the evolution of his knowledge base and ever-improving clinical results over time.

However, as someone who has had the opportunity to watch him over a ten-year period, I have witnessed the truth of this prediction in action many times. Year by year, additional layers of knowledge become more available. People who were previously not able to be healed fully are now able to be healed more completely.

Master John Douglas explains this phenomenon from his viewpoint as: "Deeper layers of pathology or pathological processes are blocked from my clairvoyant vision until Nature in her Divine Timing decides it is right to unfold another level of knowledge to the world."

This gives a whole new perspective between the relationship of scientific progress/technology and the rise of what Master John Douglas calls "world consciousness." In other words, what we are able to manifest in this world is directly related to the sum total of energies reflected in the "soup" that is measurable as "world consciousness."

While this sounds very far-fetched to the average person, and certainly complicates the equation for why specific events happen to a person, community, nation or the world as a whole, I can assure you that there is a discrete scanning frequency signal that is measurable for "world consciousness", no different from a discrete frequency signal indicating which negative life form is the root cause of a given disease state.

Furthermore, this measurement of "world consciousness", which determines the deservingness of manifesting anything on this planet at any given time, whose frequency can be directly experienced by scanning, is clearly influenced by specific events of a spiritual nature.

For example, the level of charitable giving, various manifestations of goodwill towards others, certain forms of ritualistic prayer and even the existence and measurable impact of the annual Elite Development Courses all affect this measurement known as "world consciousness."

It may surprise the reader to know that the relationship between Transcendental Meditation practiced in large groups and the manifestation of independent variables of societal conflict or harmony have all been published in indexed scientific peer-reviewed journals as part of the scientific evidence base for many decades. In other words, the influence of conscious-intention as a defined energy, focused in a defined manner (specific form of meditation) and its ability to alter independently controlled variables within society (crime rates, hospitalization rates, etc.) is a reproducible event already demonstrated in the scientific literature.[1]

[1](Hagelin JS et al. Effects of group practice of the Transcendental Meditation program on preventing violent crime in Washington, DC: results of the National Demonstration Project, June-July 1993. Social Indicators Research 1999 47:153-201

Dillbeck MC et al. Test of a field model of consciousness and social change: Transcendental Meditation and TM-Sidhi program and decreased urban crime. Journal of Mind and Behavior 1988 9:457-486)

While I am very familiar with this knowledge brought forth by Maharishi Mahesh Yogi, the founder of the TM movement, and these scientific publications documenting the positive effect of mediation on seemingly independent societal variables, I believe that this entire subject of inquiry has now evolved even further.

The insights shared by Master John Douglas regarding the cause and effect relationships, which underlie his ability to perform long-term medical remissions by miraculous healings, has revealed deeper layers of Natural Law. He has revealed why science, technology and spirituality must be reconciled with each other to truly understand medicine accurately.

It is a difficult pill to swallow that the behavior of oneself, one's family, one's ancestors, one's community, state or nation is all part of a feedback loop that determines how world consciousness plays out and how disease and misfortune manifests for each of us. The cosmic perspective needed to understand the enormity of this reality is not natural to the human condition. It is initially rejected by our subconscious, our conscious mind and our ego, which like to believe in the illusion of control. Furthermore, our societal structures and conditioning typically teach us to avoid taking personal responsibility for our actions, as it is always easier and more psychologically comfortable to blame others, be they individuals or institutions.

Yet, this failure to understand the deeper laws that govern our reality is precisely the source of the imbalance we discussed at the beginning of the book. Following the "trail of bread crumbs" suggested in this book is exactly the corrective action plan necessary to rebalance our world's precarious position with regard to world consciousness and the fate of our planet.

The corrective action plan is simple:

Know yourself. Know your God.

And, know your place in the universe.

Love yourself. Love your God. And, love your place in the universe.

Sounds simple? It is simple on one level. But, it requires some focus and discipline on another level.

17

Science, Technology and Spirituality.
The Future Junction Point of Medicine.

"The great tragedy of Science—the slaying of a beautiful hypothesis by an ugly fact." Thomas Huxley: Biologist 1870

The tragedy of science in our era is that we are deluded into thinking that we are masters of our universe. After all, we have been to the moon and back. We have unlocked the power of the atom. We have created great abundance with industrial agriculture, advanced technologies and have discovered much of the genetic code. Why then is the world such a mess? Why are we losing the heath care battle to ever mutating infectious microbes and the epidemic of chronic diseases?

The answer is that we are ignoring the ugly fact that we live in delusion. We believe that we are in control instead of the Divine being in control. Such is the hubris and conceit of mankind.

So, what is the corrective action plan? How do we jolt ourselves into facing this psychologically disturbing reality of our plight?

As always, those who fail to learn from history are doomed to repeat it. So, let's take a look back at history for some possible clues to future solutions.

In ancient times, philosophy and science were one. Granted, these were simpler times, but the great philosopher Plato had the audacity to suggest that even politics, along with both philosophy and science, should be merged as one overarching discipline to guide the Good and Correct life. Hence, his logical recommendation that society should be ruled by his "Philosopher Kings", those graduates of his elite secret school where students were taught a curriculum which included meditation, the development of innate but latent "super-powers" and self-discipline. Self-serving you might say, given his status as the premier philosopher of his time. But, was he wrong?

While our planet is much more advanced, both scientifically and technologically than in Plato's day, so too is the heightened peril of our very existence as a planet and as a species. It is my contention that all advanced societies pass through a junction point where spirituality and science/technology must reach a perfect balance. This balance is achieved when all of these subjects of inquiry exist as one discipline, as they did in Plato's time.

If this balance is successfully achieved, then the evolution of the planet and its inhabitants proceed forward to be an "advanced race", an "advanced civilization" within the many civilizations inhabiting our universe.

If this planetary balance is not achieved, we fail to do so at our great peril. The planet may be doomed to the continuation of unbalanced thinking and unbalanced actions of its inhabitants. In the worse-case scenario, it could be destroyed and join the asteroid belt of our solar system, the graveyard of our other such failed societies.

These asteroid remnants are derived, I believe, from the societies who over the millennium of time have failed the evolutionary test to balance science and technology with spirituality.

How can I make such an outlandish statement?

Because the art of "scanning", which is the foundation of how medical remissions by miraculous healing are achieved, is not merely a method to achieve healing. It can also reveal the "truth of all matter", as Master John Douglas would say.

Aside from accurately guiding the focus of healing by uncovering the root causes of many incurable diseases, the process of "scanning" opens the window of heretofore hidden laws and knowledge, which allows us to better understand the deeper truth of our sojourn as inhabitants of this planet we call Earth.

The disciplines of science, technology and spirituality can no longer be separated. To understand either, is to understand all. This is the message that so many theoretical physicists have proposed over the past few decades. They have shown us the inaccuracy of artificially and arbitrarily separating consciousness, physical reality and the quantum field states, when in reality they are different aspects of but one reality, the play and display of energy.

To be more precise, I am not invoking supernatural explanations to explain the observation that predictable, verifiable and reproducible medical remissions have been achieved by miraculous healings. Rather, as we have discussed, the power and ability to obtain such "miracles" exists latently within each of us. It just requires the proper training, discipline and practice for each of us to harness this potential and create our own "miracles."

When the universe is properly understood from this wider perspective, there is no such thing as the "supernatural." We realize that the supernatural is merely an expanded understanding of the breadth of natural law which extends past our current sciences of physics, biology, physiology, etc.

Unfortunately, our current failure to understand this breadth of natural law and the true relationship between mind, matter, and spirituality leads to a false and inaccurate scientific model. A model that does not have the ability to solve our planets many challenges. This is the very state of illusion, hubris and ignorance which we now find ourselves in as a species and as a planet.

While it is not necessary in this discussion to alter our terminology of medicine, physics and spirituality to the terminology of theology, I believe that to do so, while it may offend some, may make this material more accessible to some of our readers. Therefore, I will attempt to translate my observations and explanations into the terminology of theology as well.

From my standpoint there is no mutual exclusion. I view theological nomenclature as the personification of discrete intelligent energy fields within nature, each field fulfilling its innate role as part of the Whole.

Our current planetary imbalance, which is reflected in most human activity, is the result of a species that is advanced scientifically and technologically, without

being grounded in the reality of our Divinity. We are one of the few places in the universe where the existence of God and his celestial realm is all but forgotten.

Why does this doubt of our Divine connection even exist?

It exists because, unlike other planets and other realms of creation, where the ratio percentage of Divine energy to Demonic energy or the ratio of Positive energy to Negative energy or the ratio of Forces of Light to Forces of Darkness can be anywhere from 100% to zero % or zero % to 100%, planet Earth lives in a state of perfect duality: 50% positive energy and 50% negative energy. This is the deeper reality that controls our existence per Master John Douglas and his explanation for "why nothing is as it appears." How can it be otherwise, when 50% of all we see is Divinely constructed to delude us by design? And yet, all is perfect.

I use the word "perfect" because, while these two energies are juxtaposed, at their root both are Divine. Our theology books agree that even the dark energies of Demons are Divine. How could it not be so, if all manifestation is created by the One God, the primal force and energy of All. Again, I would assert that the "supernatural" does not exist. It is called into question only within the vacuum of ignorance about broader natural laws which have yet to be discovered and understood.

None of us, as humans, would claim to be omniscient and omnipotent. Therefore, our thinking, which is the foundation of our actions, suffers from a predictably narrow human perspective trapped in a linear representation of time and space. The universe is actually multi-dimensional and infinitely prismatic, a field of infinite correlation and infinite possibilities.

What if this larger, more cosmic perspective was open to our conscious awareness? What if each of us really has a Divine core, that with training, could be accessed, developed and blossom into a new, more evolved foundation for our thinking and actions, a foundation of conscious awareness that could account for the almost infinite variables which govern life moment to moment?

Ah yes, we have now returned back to Plato and his elite secret school to create Philosopher Kings. But that already occurred in ancient times. Look where it got us. Does a new "school" or organized body of knowledge exist to allow us as a species to rebalance ourselves, to ground our thinking and actions in a larger Divine perspective and thus provide a foundation for a more correct scientific model, a scientific model that has infinitely more power and predictability, a model able to solve the major problems facing our world?

Fortunately, I believe that the answer to this question is "yes."

It often is said that: "Within great crises exists great opportunities." There is no greater example of this than the personalized obstacle/opportunity that disease creates for all of us. We all are so busy with the mundane details of our lives that we do not take the time to understand the real nature of our existence, the deeper Divine Laws underlying our moment-to-moment reality; that is, until disease shocks us into a reevaluation of our priorities and decision-making

Disease, by its very manifestation, is testimony to a personal imbalance with the Laws of Nature. It is our personal "wake up" call. Just as the experience of "pain" is a useful signal to the body that something is "out of order", disease reminds us that no matter how smart and successful we may be in this world, we are powerless: Powerless to control our next thought; powerless to control our fate; powerless, in most cases, to even understand the root cause of our plight.

And, while this is the nature of our existence to date, our future does not have to be this way. Using the accepted tools of science to measure the validity of truth, by studying the root cause of incurable diseases, we can now revisit the mechanisms of action which create medical remissions by miraculous healing and how they occur in a predictable manner. I believe this study into the nature of medical remissions by miraculous healing, over the test of time, will hold up to rigorous scientific scrutiny.

These medical miracles occur by rediscovering our connection to Divinity, our reconnection to our own inner nature, which allow us to rebalance and work in harmony with the Laws of Nature instead of against the Laws of Nature. While this sounds like "New Age" jargon, it is really common sense.

Consider: The human physiology is not meant to be fueled by either salt water or gasoline, so to expect a good result from that diet is counter to the Laws of Nature, as it is disruptive to the design of the human body. This is to be contrasted with supplying the body with all the trace minerals, vitamins and nutritious food required to keep it functioning well, a diet in accordance with the Laws of Nature.

To unravel these deeper Laws of Nature, the understanding of which has both the power to create and explain miraculous healing, is to understand the junction point where science, technology and spirituality must be one.

Our last case study is a perfect example of the limited perspective of our current medical model, or medical paradigm, versus the reality of what can be known and corrected by accessing our Divine Nature through the process of scanning.

18

The Misdiagnosis of Marfan Syndrome as a Genetic Disease

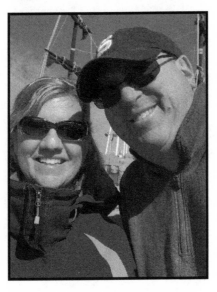

Meet Adam, a 46-year-old high school history teacher, who is very athletically inclined and who formerly coached multiple sports at his school. Adam's father, an infectious disease specialist, also had Marfan syndrome. This is not surprising given that it is currently classified as an autosomal dominant disease which means that it has a 50% chance of being passed onto your children. Adam's father, unfortunately, is now deceased from lymphoma, not from Marfan syndrome. Adam's daughter has been genetically tested and does not carry the Marfan genetic trait.

As a young child, Adam had very poor eyesight with high myopia, typical of Marfan syndrome. He has the classic Marfan appearance which is physically tall and thin, with an unusually long wingspan.

Ten years ago, while undergoing the extraction of multiple wisdom teeth, he spontaneously, without warning, had his first cardiac event and was rushed to the local emergency room where he was found to have a markedly enlarged heart due to severe regurgitation from a mostly obstructed aortic valve. He proceeded to have emergency surgery involving a complete aortic root and valve replacement with the preeminent Marfan cardiothoracic surgeon at Johns Hopkins. His cardiac status has been stable since that surgery, although he now must utilize Benicar and Metoprolol to control his systemic hypertension, Coumadin to avoid blood clots due to the valve prosthesis and utilize a C-pap machine for sleep apnea.

His surgeon explained to him that, "aortic valve failure typically happens to Marfan patients in their fifties and sixties. It was unusual for yours to fail at age 35."

While his cardiac status was stabilized postoperatively, unfortunately, Adam relates that: "I still felt like I was 60 years old." His Marfan syndrome had now affected both shoulders to the point where he was about to schedule bilateral rotator cuff surgeries. His athletically active life, both as a high school sports coach and as a high-level recreational player, disappeared. In its place, Marfan syndrome "had put me on the sidelines, more in the capacity of a nonparticipating athletic director. If I tried to do a corner kick with my girls' soccer team, or pitch to my baseball team, I would inevitably traumatize my body to the point where my joints would be swollen and painful. I was living with day to day pain of eight out of ten and had a severely reduced quality of life."

At this juncture in his life, Adam was unacquainted with Master John Douglas. Fortunately, his wife, Jen (pictured with Adam), had listened to some of the audio Health Repair tools. She convinced him to attend a seminar in Santa Fe, New Mexico.

Like many of our other case studies, Adam reported feeling "extremely serene and peaceful during the seminar and group healing session." When he drew lottery ticket #1 to see Master John as the first one-on-one session of that day, "I just had a good feeling that something special was about to happen."

During his one-on-one session, Adam reports that: "Master John nailed everything. He described my father's illness (non-Marfan related) and other details that he could not have possibly known."

Adam describes his session as: "I was very locked-in and symbiotic with Master John. My body was tingling all over with a sensation that is hard to describe." At the end of the session, "I felt way different, ten years younger. I was actually able to raise my arms and give him a hug." Pre-session, raising his arms to that degree had been impossible.

The day following the session with Master John Douglas, Adam reported: "My Fitbit showed that I walked 22,000 steps that day, when formerly my limit would have been 6,000 steps. I no longer had the shortness of breath that would limit my activity. I no longer felt the extreme tiredness that would force me to take a nap in the middle of the day."

Since that healing session with Master John Douglas, which occurred on May 22, 2016, Adam's chronic pain and shortness of breath has never returned. He reports being able to resume full age-appropriate activity once again. "Sure, I will feel routine aches and pains if I overdo it athletically, but I can still hang in there for three sets with my daughter who is on the high school tennis team. My energy level has returned to normal and I lead a very active life at both work and play."

Adam reports: "I have never had to follow through with the anticipated rotator cuff surgeries, much to the surprise of my orthopedic surgeons, who are unable to explain why I am better." Adam further reports: "At my annual cardiology exam, I exceeded expectations and was subsequently released from my annual participation in the Johns Hopkins Marfan cardiac study."

Although he has never attended another Master John Douglas seminar since his healing in 2016, he reports that: "I feel like he looks in on me from time to time. I wish that I could just run into him on the street and say hi. I feel very blessed and think the world of him."

What is even more remarkable than the instantaneous reversal of all chronic clinical limitations which were leading to inevitable surgery is that in this case study we see that a presumed genetic disease is "cured" once the underlying infection is identified and eradicated.

Master John Douglas discovered, using his clairvoyant vision, that Marfan syndrome is actually caused by a nano-bacteria living in the soft tissues and joints. The classical clinical signs of Marfan syndrome are actually secondary side effects created by the infectious nano-bacteria, which create dehydration of the infected tissues and a resulting flaking away of tissue integrity.

During the personal one-on-one session, Master John Douglas was able to go back in time and scan Adam's father's physiology for the existence of the same nano-bacteria now affecting his son. As the same nano-bacteria was found to be present in his father's physiology, the root cause of this disease now must be understood as infectious, although it mimics a hereditary disease. What is inherited is the immune systems susceptibility to be infected with this specific infectious organism, not the disease itself.

Once again, we see the limitations of having the wrong medical paradigm. As conventional medicine lacks the key information and evidence regarding the infectious etiology of this disease, our existing paradigm leads to the wrong conclusion; namely, that this disease is genetic and incurable.

In our current medical paradigm, all we can offer are surgical interventions, which to be fair, are life-saving, just as his emergency valve replacement was life-saving. And while saving one's life is nothing to sneeze at, why not cure this "incurable" disease by understanding its root cause? Why treat it at the level of the symptoms, when we can treat it at the level of the cause?

A wise man once told me: "Never solve the problem on the level of the problem. Solve the problem at the deepest possible level." The analogy is, why paint the leaves green on a tree which is struggling, when watering the root will return it to health.

In this case, Master John Douglas certainly could not have performed life-saving cardiac surgery. He has no medical training, let alone cardiothoracic specialty surgical training. But he does have full access to the frequency of all particles in creation. By listening to that song, he was able to cure this "incurable" disease. Increased knowledge is increased power.

At this point, I hopefully have painted a picture of where we are as a planet and what we can achieve if we "play our cards right."

While I don't wish to repeat myself, the following disclaimer given at the start of the book is important enough to repeat one more time:

To aid with the launch of this book and the dissemination of this knowledge, a not for profit LLC charitable foundation has been formed: The STS Foundation. STS is short for science, technology and spirituality. **I am but a spokesman on behalf of the foundation and again wish to remind the reader that my words are not to be taken as medical advice from a physician. Rather, my words are to be taken from the perspective of a medically trained observer, vouching for the validity and reproducibility of this specific opportunity for faith-based healing via the knowledge presented by Master John Douglas, and adopted by the**

Church of the Master Angels.

This brings up one final point. How does one reconcile this knowledge with one's own religious beliefs or scientific training?

A few targeted questions and answers that were raised by the multiple editors who helped work on this book may shed additional intellectual light and emotional comfort to these sensitive questions.

QUESTIONS AND ANSWERS

Question #1: It's one thing to claim that everything is composed of frequency and quite another to say that we can be aware of all of these. That a person can be aware of all of these from the entire universe at once seems very implausible. That we can be aware of some types of such frequencies or such frequencies as are located somewhere in someone's body, seems plausible. The former requires a kind of omniscience which I doubt Master John Douglas claims to have. How do we reconcile these ideas?

Answer #1: It is correct that it is beyond the capability of the human central nervous system to exhibit the properties of omniscience or omnipotence that seemingly are required to perform various healings or miracles. That is why I joke that our claim to fame as an Elite Course Graduate is not that we personally perform miracles, because we do not. All miracles are performed by the Master Healing Angels. Elite Graduates have been given a hot line to the angelic kingdom to ask for help. We ask, they do the actual healing.

The Master Healing Angels do not have human nervous systems. They have divine nervous systems. By their very nature, by their multi-pointed and multi-dimensional prismatic awareness, they are capable of simultaneous perceptions of all things. We as humans are not. We cannot know all things in the universe simultaneously. We simply do not have the "hardware or software" to be aware of all things simultaneously.

I would, however, put Master John into a different category than the rest of us humans. If, as I contend, he is the incarnation of a Celestial Being whose abilities grow as world consciousness allows, then his nervous system is constructed in a very different fashion from the rest of the human race. He is in a process of reverse evolution, angelic to human, while we are in a process of ascension, human to angelic. As such, the abilities inherent within his nervous system in no way resemble our abilities, even with the advanced training received at the Elite Development Course. This is one example where the student will not surpass the teacher.

Question #2: I am wary of the claims about the pineal gland's involvement. This is not because I know it is not involved but because I don't know that it is involved. No evidence is given that it is involved. I think that unless John's brain has been imaged, and imaged while he engages in healing, so that pineal gland involvement can be established, it is better to leave open the discussion of what goes on when healing occurs. This appeal to pineal gland involvement was something Descartes made with no good basis. I don't think that you or Master John should do so unless you have some pretty good evidence for such.

Answer #2: While I hesitate to venture into assertions that have no current scientific proof, discussions regarding the pineal gland are still of interest, both from an historical perspective and from my direct experience on the level of awareness as an Elite Course Graduate.

From an historical perspective, the seventeenth century philosopher and scientist Rene Descartes believed the human pineal gland to be the "principle seat of the soul and the place where all our thoughts are formed." He believed that the pineal gland "was the junction point between the body and the soul."

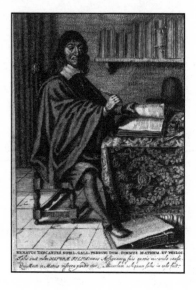

In the late nineteenth century, Madame Blavatsky, who co-founded the Theosophy Society, identified the pineal gland with the Hindu concept of the third eye or the Anja chakra. This is still a widely held belief within current spiritual literature. Blavatsky, who studied in Tibet, described Theosophy as "the synthesis of science, religion and philosophy."

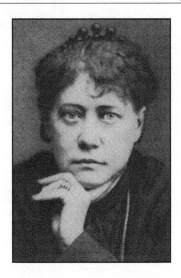

It is entirely possible that our failure to scientifically demonstrate any unique capabilities of this gland, beyond the known endocrine functions involving melatonin, is not because it has no additional capabilities but because these functions are only seen on the level of the more, subtle energy bodies which are not the domain yet of modern science. It is entirely possible that as technology develops, that we will be able to verify additional functions of this endocrine gland and prove or disprove these more esoteric assertions. Until then, I am not uncomfortable citing these historical claims, with the caveat that I will continue to suspend scientific judgement until a later date.

On a more personal level, from the subjective level of my awareness, I have noticed a profound change in the inner mental image of how my pineal gland functions since taking the Elite Development Course. In my mind's eye, this gland formerly functioned like a broken black and white television with lots of static, whereas now it appears as a high-speed computer open to the knowledge cloud of all possibilities. Imagination? Perhaps. I eagerly await the day when our technology develops to the point where this discussion can be put to more objective rigorous testing.

Question #3: Please describe the learning process involved with scanning in more detail both for Master John Douglas and for Elite Course participants.

Answer #3: I once heard Master John joking about how easy we have it compared to him with regards to our learning curve to develop our scanning abilities. Master John reports: "I did not have a human mentor, only angelic mentors." He relates that all of his early learning was a process of trial and error, where "the angels would mildly electrocute me to signal to me that I had the wrong answer."

I am happy to report that the Elite Development Course participants learn in a group setting, where they can take advantage of checking their scanning accuracy against more advanced scanners, who have done this for a while. It typically requires approximately 10,000 scans to become proficient in the accuracy of one's scanning abilities. We jokingly call this the "100 challenge." After graduation from the Elite Development Course, do 100 scans a day for 100 days and you have reached the goal of 10,000 scans.

Question #4: Have other medical doctors and health professionals peer reviewed the material presented in this book, similar to the review process that was needed for your publications in the various medical journals (previously published articles are found by hitting the "research" tab at the top of the home page at www. masterangels.org)

Answer #4: The typical peer-review process implemented when submitting to the various medical journals is slightly different, in that the reviewers remain anonymous to the author. The author then modifies his submission to meet the objections of the various reviewers in the hope that the revised edits have satisfied their objections. If the edits achieve this goal, then the resubmitted article receives approval and is published.

The process of peer review undertaken for this book was different in that the medical doctors and other health professionals who were asked to review the material were not anonymous. In fact, they were my true peers in that they all have graduated from the Elite Development Course. In most cases, they actually had first-hand knowledge of the case study subjects pre/post medical remissions and miraculous healings, as they have followed many of them for multiple years. While this certainly introduces some bias to the review process, I believe the positives of their concrete personal experience and direct knowledge of many of the subjects herein reported outweigh the potential negatives.

Question #5: While the book is written, for the most part, in the jargon of science and medical terminology, how do you rectify all of this discussion of the angelic world, which is clearly not an ordinary subject of science?

Answer #5: This is a very legitimate question and deserves a multilayered answer. Historically, humans have reported seeing or communicating with angels for many millennia over many geographies, societies and religions. I take the existence of these historical reports as a single piece of evidence, no different than the reports of herbal medical cures which have existed in other cultures for thousands of years. Modern medicine and science are just now beginning to recognize the healing powers of various traditional herbal botanicals, as well as meditation, yoga, tai chi, chi gong, etc. But until recently, these practices were thought to be merely folly or placebo. The growing scientific evidence base on these mind/body practices now attest to their legitimacy.

Many of the Elite Development Course graduates have some level of celestial perception, whereby their enhanced senses allow for direct communication (sight/auditory/ mental imagery) with the Master Healing Angels. Kathryn's case study and her description of her angelic communications both before and after her heart attack, are a perfect example of this phenomena.

Again, to use an historical analogy, infectious microbes existed well before the discovery of the microscope. Yet, before the invention of the microscope those physicians who believed in the germ theory were subject to ridicule. It is unclear to me how close we are to having the technology to provide external objective verification of all of the occult infectious life forms which are the root cause of many of our "incurable diseases" and of the angelic kingdom and their direct relationship to the healing process.

However, as I previously stated in the published peer reviewed articles, I believe the day will come when yet-to-be-discovered enhanced technology reveals the existence of all of the variables we have discussed. Until then, I am comfortable suspending judgement as to their external scientific verification and suggest that we all continue to enjoy the benefits of miraculous healing and long-term remissions that are clearly reproducible.

As a final thought, there are many levels of scientific evidence and testing for validity. Each level, e.g. corroborated observation versus DNA analysis versus understanding mechanisms of action versus satisfaction surveys, has merit in and of itself. The failure to provide evidence on each level does not, in and of itself, invalidate the evidence already established.

Question #6: With all this discussion of "curing incurable diseases", are the Elite Course Development graduates actually practicing medicine without a license?

Answer #6: The answer to this question is an emphatic NO for many reasons. The most important reason is that the actual healing is accomplished by invoking the Master Healing Angels to help a person with whatever difficulty in life they are challenged with. As neither prayer nor contacting angels for help is within the domain of medicine at this point in time, if Elite Development Course graduates are guilty of practicing medicine, then every Minister, Rabbi, Chaplain and Reverend are all guilty of the same charge.

Question #7: How do you reconcile the fact that you seem to give credit for a miraculous healing to case studies who ultimately relapse?

Answer #7: I use the term "miraculous healing" to denote a change of events in the natural course of a disease which is otherwise unexplainable, especially when the root cause of the disease is known, and the cure is created by direct intention. The ability to reproduce this event for the same disease state by multiple healers only increases our confidence in this scientific reality.

Let's reexamine our case study involving Dana, who had a prosthetic joint infection, which left untreated with surgery or antibiotics, would have a high probability of sepsis or death. Yet, after a direct intervention by Master John Douglas to identify and kill the root cause of the infection, also witnessed in real-time by myself, the anticipated untreated result of sepsis or death, did not occur. In fact, the patient actually thrived for many months.

I know of no other way to describe this event, as I could clearly witness the frequency emanating from the infectious organism totally disappear after Master John's direct intention to kill the infectious organism. The fact that ultimately this case study went on to have additional surgery and intravenous antibiotics eight months later does not diminish, in my opinion, the remission and miraculous healing of the initial life-threatening event.

I would assert that the same reasoning is true for Ann,

who had metastatic squamous cell carcinoma, already presented in Chapter 5. To document the remission of a stage four cancer where the patient could actually "see" on the level of her awareness the transformation of her physiology from a pathologic state to a healthy state and to corroborate her subjective experience with objective radiology scans meets my criteria of a miracle, regardless of whether or not she had a reoccurrence many years later.

To state the obvious, we will all die at some point in time, whether we first receive a miracle or not prior to our death. To fail to appreciate a miracle once received, because of a later change in one's health, is to not appreciate an event of Divine Intervention. Ultimately this is, in my opinion, a cosmic tragedy.

Question #8: If, as you say, the real healers are the Master Healing Angels and not the Elite Development Course graduates, why can't the average person in the street just achieve the same results now that we know to direct our prayers to the Master Healing Angels?

Answer #8: Remember that I used the analogy of obtaining new software and new hardware to upgrade our present state human nervous system towards a more celestial nervous system, which is capable of communicating more easily with the celestial realm. To continue the analogy, these upgrades accelerate the Elite Graduate from "dial-up" service to fiber optic service in our ability to communicate with the celestial realm. This upgrade is achieved by attending the Elite Development Course.

Theoretically, although it is more cumbersome, it is completely possible that an individual without attending the Elite Development Course can communicate with the Master Healing Angels and request a miraculous healing. Some evidence of the truth of this phenomenon is that prior to attending the Elite Development Course many of the Elite Development Course attendees have reported having seen Celestial Beings in their dreams which closely resemble the Master Healing Angels, as they are depicted within the Elite Development Course material.

None the less, the likelihood of developing a predictable and functional relationship with this realm of Celestial Beings is greatly enhanced by the physiological and spiritual upgrades and empowerments experienced within the Elite Development Course curriculum. To use the jargon of theology, one's worthiness and deservingness are elevated to facilitate the possibility of this relationship.

Question #9: How do you answer the question as to why these hidden, unknown infectious life forms are not seen with all of the medical technology at our disposal, i.e. electron microscopy, virology, microbiology, parasitology, etc.?

Answer #9: From an historical perspective, even in a disease as recent as the discovery of AIDS in the late 1970s, if you don't know what you are looking for, your filters to find it may prohibit its discovery. Even today, DNA confirmation of an infectious entity requires that the tissue sample be accessible and that we know which DNA marker we are looking for. For current context, the bacterial DNA load or microbiome of our digestive tract is greater than the sum total of our own DNA. So, isolating which of the microbiome DNA is the pathologic root cause of an undiscovered disease is like looking for a needle in a haystack. This dilemma is still in effect even with the technology of a scanning electron microscopy which has resolution to the Nano-particle level.

Developing technologies such as dark field microscopy, and live blood cell analysis, may provide future insights into this hidden world but these techniques are still being scientifically validated.

To further complicate matters, we have not even discussed how portals or worm holes exist connecting parallel universes, and how infectious agents literally pop in and out of our present space/time continuum. Just imagine the difficulty of imaging something as it travels momentarily through these time/space anomalies. These more complex variables will be discussed in more detail in Medical Miracles book 2 at some future date.

Question #10: I hate even to ask this question, but how do you reconcile the knowledge contained in this book and what is taught at the Elite Development Course, for a fundamentalist Christian?

Answer #10: As you know, I have tried to explain the material in this book within the historical context of my attempt to make scientific and intellectual sense of the many hundreds and thousands of miracles which I have observed either directly or indirectly over the past ten years. Additionally, to make this material more accessible to readers who prefer using the terminology of theology, versus science, I have attempted to translate and integrate the terminologies between these two viewpoints.

As I said in the Introduction, our future as a planet depends on us coming to an understanding that science, technology, and spirituality must be understood as one all-encompassing Truth. Knowledge is knowledge. Knowledge is not owned by anyone.

But more to your point, I do not believe that neither Master John Douglas nor the Elite Development Course, teaches anything that would give pause to a fundamentalist Christian. In fact, within the Church of the Master Angels is a beautiful stained-glass window depicting Jesus, which was donated by a Christian family from Texas. Both the husband and wife who made this donation, and members of their family, attend the Elite Development Courses each year to further enhance their knowledge. So, clearly, they are not offended, nor feel their religious beliefs are compromised, in any way.

There is also a religious icon which is only revealed to Elite Development Course participants, as part of the course curriculum. While I cannot discuss this icon in detail, I will reveal that it illustrates a hierarchy of how the universe is organized from the earthly structures of this world to the highest realms of the heavens. There is no hierarchical representation of anything higher than Jesus depicted in this icon. So, hopefully that will ease your mind.

On a personal note, while it is true that I am a man of science and have no advanced training in theology or seminary degrees, all I can tell you is that I do my best every day to live my life in a state of innocence, surrender and faith to the one and only Lord our God. It is my sincere hope that the knowledge contained in this book helps anyone who reads it achieve greater faith, surrender and homage.

To quote another wise man I know: "There are only two important things in life. One, ask for help. And two, be grateful when it is received."

DISCLAIMER

This book was authored and prepared by Richard L. Sarnat M.D., in his personal capacity. The opinions and views expressed herein are his own. They do not purport to reflect, and are not authorized to be stated as, the opinions or views of CMA International Foundation, d/b/a Church of the Master Angels (a Delaware not-for-profit organization), Global S.E.L.F. Foundation (an Illinois not-for-profit organization) or any of their Directors, Officers, members, agents, representatives and/or employees.

Made in the USA
San Bernardino, CA
10 March 2020